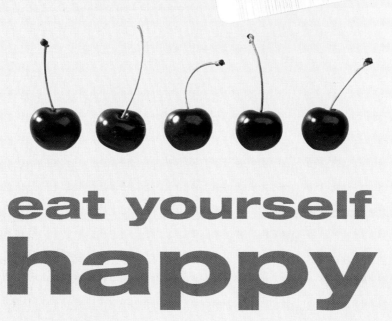

eat yourself
happy

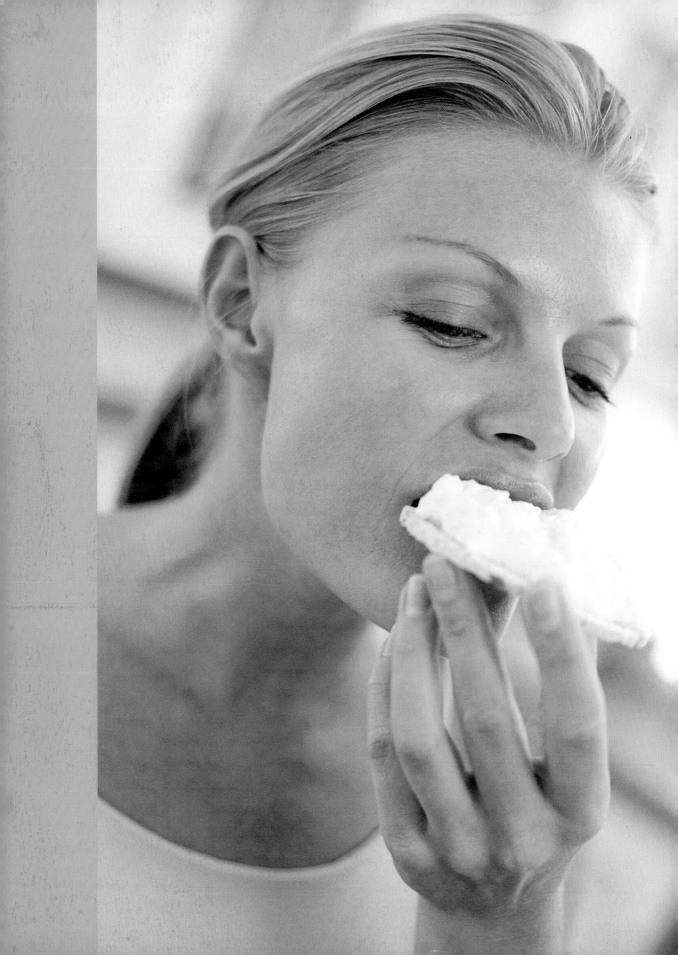

eat yourself
happy

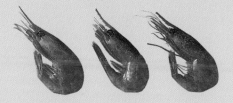

Nutrients, foods
and recipes for optimal
mental health

DR. MICHAEL T. ISAAC & DR. MARIA B. ISAAC

CARROLL & BROWN PUBLISHERS LIMITED

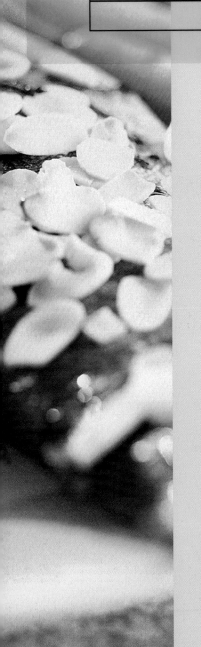

First published in 2004 in the United Kingdom by

Carroll & Brown Publishers Limited
20 Lonsdale Road
London NW6 6RD

Project Editor Ian Wood
Art Editors Emily Cook, Anne Fisher
Photographer Jules Selmes

A CIP catalogue record for this book is available from the British Library

ISBN 1-903258-82-0

10987654321

Reproduced by RALI, Spain
Printed and bound in Italy by MS Printing

The information contained in this book should be used as a
general reference guide and does not constitute, and is not
intended to substitute for, an expert's medical or legal advice.
Not all the drugs listed here are available in all countries and,
even if they are available, may not be licensed for the
purpose given in this book. You should always consult your
doctor, healthcare professional or pharmacist if in any doubt.

CONTENTS

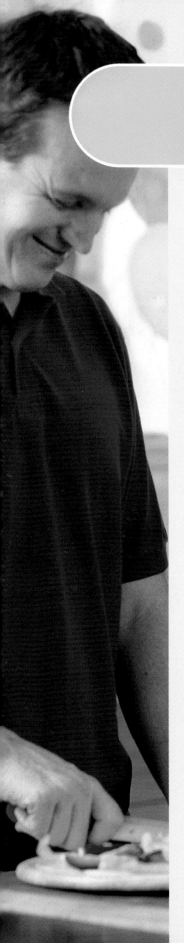

INTRODUCTION

More than at any time in history, people in the developed world now look to the food they eat not simply to keep them alive, but also to keep them healthy. In growing numbers, people are rejecting "artificial", chemically enhanced, or synthetic foods in favour of "natural", healthy, or organic products. More people are buying "functional foods"—such as probiotic yoghurt drinks—that are supposed to aid health.

Cutting through the hype

Beliefs that certain foods or certain diets promote health are thousands of years old. What has changed is that it is now commonplace to find not only organic food, but also food supplements, vitamins, minerals, amino acids and a host of other products in supermarkets and health food stores. Big claims are made for these products. The right food, and the right supplements, can keep you healthy and even, they say, cure you of disease. But how much of this is based on evidence, and how much is simply hype? How can we decide among competing claims in such a valuable market? If you take all the advice, follow all the diets, and down the daily doses of vitamins and supplements as recommended, you might rattle as you walk, but will you live any longer, or be significantly healthier in body or mind?

In some countries it is against the law to claim that a food or supplement can cure or prevent a disease. This is mainly to help ensure that people do not ignore the symptoms of an underlying disease by trying to cure themselves with food. But some foods do prevent disease. A good example is folic acid supplements which, when taken by pregnant women, can prevent spina bifida in babies. So while health claims may be acceptable, medicinal claims—foods as medicines—are generally not.

Food labelling

Most people accept that eating properly can help their physical health. Recent large-scale changes in food labelling at least give people a chance to find out what is in the food they are eating. It has recently been decided in the United States, for example, that foods containing so-called trans fats must be labelled as such, and the food industry has been given notice that this will become law.

Furthermore, in a way that would have been difficult to foresee a few years ago, large players in the food industry have altered their approach to encourage healthier diets. This may in part be a protective measure against future legal action, but it also may reflect the changes of attitude within society, where consumers are beginning to demand healthier food.

Information, however, is of very little use unless you know how to interpret it. While it is all very well seeing a list of food components, unless you have some idea of what is or is not important, then you are just as susceptible to hype as if the information were not present.

Diet and mental health

With most of the current focus on diet and physical health, diet and mental health has attracted comparatively little attention until recently. This, too, has changed dramatically over recent years, and it is now widely accepted that diet can help in psychological conditions such as stress and anxiety. As practising clinical psychiatrists, we see patients who suffer from conditions as diverse as stress and mild anxiety to severely disabling schizophrenia. Many of our patients suffer from depression and other mood disorders. Our aim is to help our patients and to try to help them help themselves. Sometimes people need medication to treat the worst of their symptoms. However, treatment is not simply about taking medication or following certain exercises, it also can require changes in habits and lifestyle and, particularly, diet.

We have become convinced that anyone can improve both their mental and physical health by eating the right foods and using, judiciously, the right food supplements. We have also become convinced that there is a major gap between belief and reality when it comes to eating for mental health. Many people are put off eating healthily because they think it involves boring and tasteless food that is difficult and time-consuming to prepare, and is expensive. We hope to show that this is untrue.

The conflicting claims of diets and supplements make it difficult to know what to do for the best. In this book, we hope to trace a path through this maze and make practical suggestions, including recipes, about how you can improve your mental wellbeing through diet.

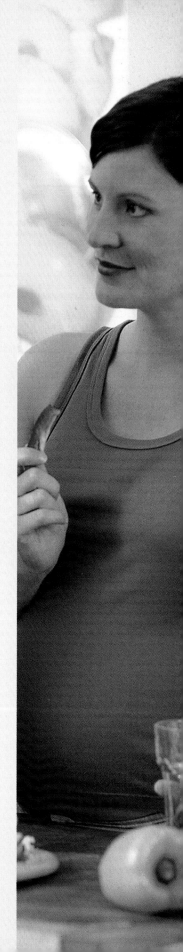

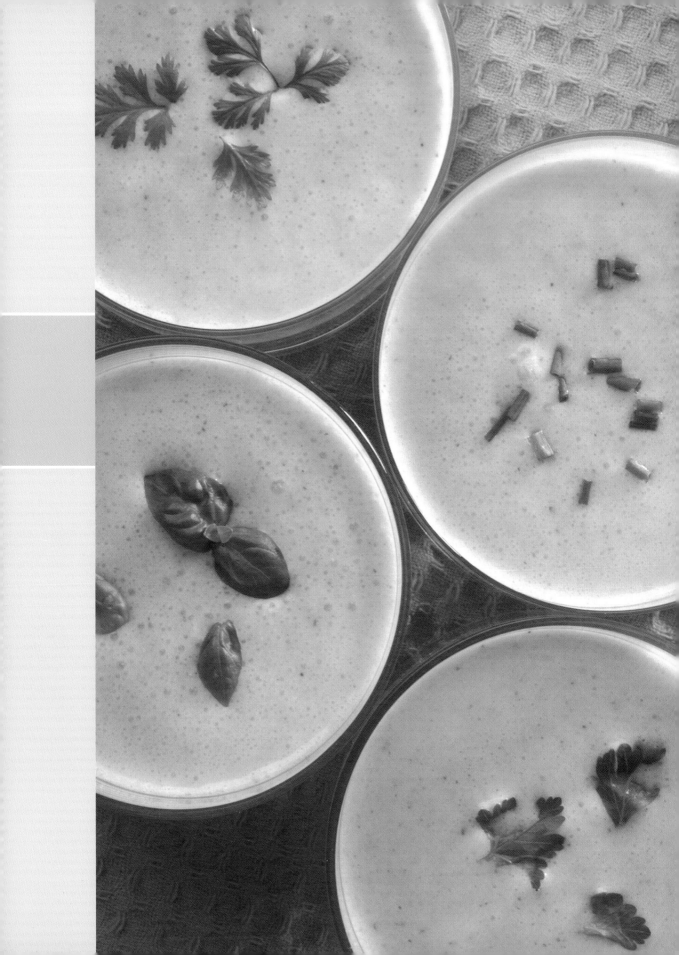

1

THE CHEMISTRY OF MOOD

brain basics

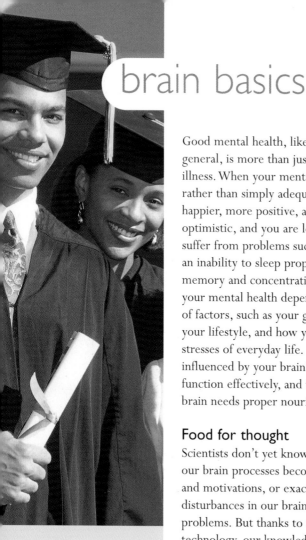

Good mental health, like good health in general, is more than just an absence of illness. When your mental health is good, rather than simply adequate, you feel happier, more positive, and more optimistic, and you are less likely to suffer from problems such as moodiness, an inability to sleep properly, or poor memory and concentration. The state of your mental health depends on a number of factors, such as your genetic make-up, your lifestyle, and how you cope with the stresses of everyday life. But it is also influenced by your brain's ability to function effectively, and to do that your brain needs proper nourishment.

Food for thought

Scientists don't yet know precisely how our brain processes become our thoughts and motivations, or exactly how chemical disturbances in our brains give rise to problems. But thanks to modern technology, our knowledge of how the brain works and how it can go wrong has increased greatly over the past ten years. And it turns out that traditional ideas about certain foods being "good for the brain" may have more than a grain of truth in them.

Like any other organ in your body, your brain needs nutrients such as proteins, fats, vitamins and minerals to maintain and repair itself, and glucose to provide the energy that powers it. It also needs the substances that it uses to make neurotransmitters, the chemicals that carry the signals between its neurons (see box, opposite). It gets all these nutrients from the food you eat, so if your diet is lacking in any of them your brain may not be able to perform at its best.

Neurons

Everything you think, feel and do depends on the activities of the billions of nerve cells packed into your brain. These nerve cells, called neurons, act as information processors. They use electrical and chemical signals to communicate with each other and with other parts of the body, and they are linked together like the components of complex electronic circuits. These circuits, which handle the many functions of your brain such as perception, thought, memory and emotions, can be tiny (involving only a few cells) or very large, covering whole regions of the brain.

Neurotransmitters

There are dozens of chemicals that act as neurotransmitters in the brain. The functions of all of them are not yet clear, but a handful of them—acetylcholine, amino acids, serotonin, noradrenaline (norepinephrine), and dopamine—make a major impact on the brain and on mental function. Many other chemicals, mainly hormones, affect the way in which the neurons work together, so they also play an important part in maintaining good mental health.

The first neurotransmitter to be identified was acetylcholine, which is widespread in the brain and in the muscles. Neurons using acetylcholine (the cholinergic neurons) play an important part in memory, and drugs that have been developed to help conditions such as Alzheimer's disease are targeted at them.

The amino acids that play an important role in brain function include glutamine, glycine, and aspartate, which

sending signals

There are about ten billion neurons in the human brain, an almost meaninglessly large number but one that pales into insignificance beside the 60 trillion junctions between them. These vast numbers of interconnected neurons and synapses, and the streams of signals that pass through them, are what gives the brain its massive information-processing power. For this processing power to function efficiently, however, it is necessary for the brain to be supplied with the correct type and amount of critical amino acids. What we eat is critical; a diet rich in essential nutrients can supply us with all the necessary amino acids or, if there is a chemical imbalance in the brain, can help to correct it. A poor diet, or one that contains too much alcohol, caffeine, or sugar, can interfere with the levels of amino acids and thus with the effective functioning of neurotransmitters, and ultimately with how well we think, remember, and carry out normal activities.

1 A neuron receives an electrical signal that causes its vesicles (clear balls) to burst.

2 Neurotransmitters such as serotonin (small dark balls) are released.

3 These cross the synaptic gap to the next neuron and bind to its receptors (yellow tees).

4 When enough serotonin is present, reuptake receptors on first neuron (orange and red tubes) stop further release.

are called excitatory neurotransmitters because they stimulate neuron activity. Another amino acid, gamma aminobutyric acid (GABA), is called an inhibitory neurotransmitter because it acts as a kind of brake to slow or shut down the activity of neurons. Several drugs important in neurology and psychiatry, including benzodiazepine tranquillizers (such as Valium), some antiepileptic drugs, and alcohol, act on the GABA system.

Serotonin (5HT, 5-hydroxy tryptamine), noradrenaline, and dopamine are the "Big Three" neurotransmitters in psychiatry, especially in mood disorders and more severe mental illnesses such as schizophrenia.

Serotonin is formed from the amino acid tryptophan, while dopamine and noradrenaline are formed from the amino acid phenylalanine. These chemicals play central roles in many brain functions, and important psychiatric drugs, including the antidepressants and antipsychotic drugs, target these chemicals.

Although neurotransmitters play such an indispensable role in the function of the brain, they are small and simple molecules, derived from substances occurring naturally in the diet. We are what we eat!

serotonin the body's happy chemical

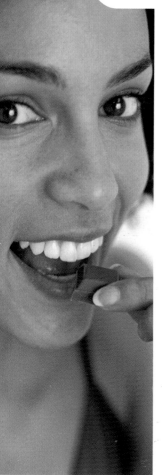

Most people have heard of the neurotransmitter serotonin. You may have read, for instance, that it is important to mood, and that eating chocolate may boost its levels. The "story" of serotonin is central to our current understanding of mood, and also of a wide range of normal brain functions, such as sleep, ageing, eating patterns, biorhythms and pain perception, and abnormal mental conditions such as anxiety, stress, post-traumatic stress, migraine, sexual disorders, schizophrenia, and addictions.

The building blocks of serotonin

Only about 1–2 percent of the body's serotonin is in the brain; the rest occurs all over the body where it has many functions, such as maintaining the flow of blood to tissues and organs, coordinating the passage of food through the bowel, and blood clotting, among others.

Serotonin cannot cross into the brain, so the brain must manufacture its own. It makes no difference if a food is rich in serotonin—none of it will get through to the brain. What matters is whether the

increasing serotonin levels

When serotonin levels are low you may be prescribed an antidepressant, as increasing serotonin in the brain is a fundamental mechanism of antidepressant action. In particular, the selective serotonin reuptake inhibitor (SSRI) class of antidepressants includes some of the most commonly prescribed drugs on the planet. These include sertraline (Zoloft, Lustral), fluoxetine (Prozac), paroxetine (Paxil, Seroxat), citalopram (Celexa, Cipramil), escitalopram (Lexapro, Cipralex), and fluvoxamine (Luvox, Faverin).

1 SINGLE SUGARS (monosaccharides) —mainly glucose—are formed when carbohydrates are broken down as part of the digestive process and absorbed into the blood.

2 INSULIN produced by the pancreas increases to cope with the rise in blood levels of glucose.

3 TRYPTOPHAN levels increase due to the higher level of insulin in the blood.

4 THE BRAIN converts its tryptophan to the neurotransmitter (brain messenger) serotonin.

food you eat contains the amino acid tryptophan, from which your brain can make serotonin. Tryptophan in food is absorbed from the stomach and intestine and crosses into the brain, where specific "serotonergic" cells, deep within the brain, use the enzyme tryptophan 5-hydroxylase to make 5-hydroxy tryptophan (5HTP). This is converted to serotonin (5-hydroxy tryptamine, 5HT).

Virtually all our tryptophan comes from the diet, and so eating foods that are rich in tryptophan can boost serotonin levels (see box). Tryptophan is taken up actively into the brain by a carrier protein that also transports other amino acids, which compete with tryptophan. Thus the brain's uptake of tryptophan (and the production of serotonin), depends not only on the tryptophan, but also on the general amino acid content of the food.

Eating carbohydrates may enhance the uptake of tryptophan. This is because insulin, the hormone that promotes the absorption of sugars, proteins and amino acids from the intestines and into cells, is especially stimulated by carbohydrates. If insulin is increased, tryptophan uptake is enhanced. This may be one reason why the sugar in a chocolate bar can provide a quick boost in mood.

The physiology of serotonin

Serotonin is a small molecule but it has extensive effects because it interacts with a rich variety of specialized proteins— serotonin (5HT) receptors—that cause cells to behave in different ways. Scientists have identified 13 subtypes of serotonin receptor, but do not yet know how they all work. The serotonin system does not work in isolation. Other neurotransmitter systems, especially the noradrenaline and dopamine systems, play roles in brain function, including mood and motivation.

good sources of tryptophan

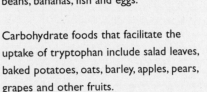

FOODS
Those high in tryptophan include turkey, milk (soy and cow or goat), cottage cheese, pecan nuts, peanuts, sunflower seeds, peas, beans, bananas, fish and eggs.

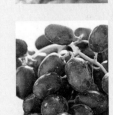

Carbohydrate foods that facilitate the uptake of tryptophan include salad leaves, baked potatoes, oats, barley, apples, pears, grapes and other fruits.

SUPPLEMENTS
Nobody knows quite how much tryptophan should supplement the diet if serotonin is low. The consensus seems to be that low mood or dysphoria requires about 1 gram per day of tryptophan in the diet, and that depression probably requires about 3 grams per day. L-tryptophan, formerly available as a supplement and used as an antidepressant, is now restricted in

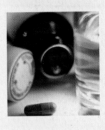

some countries. This is because of deaths from eosinophilic myalgia syndrome in people taking the synthetic compound. There is research evidence that 5-hydroxy tryptophan (5HTP), the intermediate step between tryptophan and serotonin, may be an acceptable substitute.

CLINICAL CASEBOOK
TRYPTOPHAN AND DEPRESSION

If volunteers with depression, and who are currently symptom-free, take a special drink containing amino acids, except tryptophan, their symptoms often start to come back within a few hours and they become depressed. This is reversed if they take tryptophan. Even serotonin-depleted people not suffering from depression may be less able to make decisions, especially involving the assessment of gain versus risk. They do not become depressed, but their impaired decision-making is a factor shared by depressed people.

melatonin setting your body clock

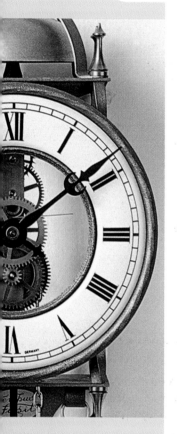

At night, the pineal gland within your brain converts serotonin into melatonin, a hormone that induces sleep. As well as helping you get to sleep, melatonin helps to reset your body's "internal clock" to keep it in step with the natural cycle of night and day. But technology allows us to pretend that we are not bound by the natural rhythms of life. For example, electric light frees us from the bondage of sunrise and sunset, and air conditioning and central heating can maintain a constant temperature. The trouble is that our bodies have not quite caught up, and they still respond to the natural cycles of night and day and the changing seasons.

This clash between our bodies' natural rhythms and our ability to ignore them becomes most evident when we disrupt them by working night shifts, or by travelling across time zones and suffering "jet lag". Such activities keep us awake and active when our brains and bodies are programmed for sleep, leading to problems such as fatigue, loss of concentration and impaired memory.

Day to night

The levels of many of the body's chemicals, including neurotransmitters and hormones, vary regularly during the day as if under the control of an internal clock. This clock is approximately synchronized with the 24-hour cycle of day and night, and uses the onset of darkness and the coming of daylight as timing cues to help keep itself in step with the outside world.

A key part of the body's internal clock mechanism is the pineal gland, a structure about the size and shape of an olive that lies deep within the brain. In the 17th century, people thought that the pineal gland was the seat of the soul, and for some religions it is the "third eye" that enables us to see beyond the physical world and into the spiritual.

During daylight, the pineal contains a high concentration of serotonin (which it makes from tryptophan), plus a small amount of melatonin. But when darkness falls, nerve signals from the eyes trigger a change in the activity of the pineal, which begins converting most of its serotonin into melatonin and slowly releasing it into the bloodstream. When daylight returns, the production of melatonin drops again. One of the main effects of the increased melatonin in the blood-

did you know?

As well as responding to the pattern of day and night, the pineal gland responds to changing daylight length as the seasons change. This leads to an increase in melatonin levels in the dark days of winter, and in some people this can cause mood disorders. Natural light therapy, which uses bright electric lamps that produce light similar to natural daylight, can help some mood disorders, including depression and so-called seasonal affective disorder (SAD), by creating artificial daylight that limits melatonin production.

stream is to induce sleep by reducing the production of the neurotransmitter dopamine (see page 16), which helps keep the brain awake and alert.

Because of its effects on sleep, melatonin is supposed to help sleep problems in depression and in Alzheimer's disease. Some say it also mitigates stress, by reducing major swings in stress hormones (corticosteroids), and it has a great reputation for treating jet lag.

Time travel

When you travel from one time zone to another, your internal body clock takes a while to synchronize itself, and it can take as much as 24 hours to recover from every time zone you cross. So it can take you a day to recover from jet lag after a flight from London to Madrid, and eight days to adjust after a flight from Los Angeles to London.

Many people take melatonin to help their body clocks reset themselves more quickly after long flights. The effectiveness of melatonin for jet lag is not universally accepted by doctors—there have been relatively few large-scale trials of the treatment—but taking 3 to 5 mg of melatonin before bedtime, and again when you wake in the middle of the night, seems to reduce and even abolish the symptoms of jet lag (tiredness, confusion, headaches and broken sleep).

There is also some evidence that melatonin in small doses (0.5 mg) can be helpful to some shift workers whose sleep rhythms are disrupted. This is not a licensed treatment, though, and if you are in any doubt, talk to your doctor before taking the supplement. The use of melatonin to combat ageing or cancer, or as an antidepressant, rests on flimsy evidence so far and we cannot recommend it.

good sources of melatonin

Oats, rice, ginger, tomatoes and bananas are especially good dietary sources of the hormone melatonin. Because it comes from serotonin, which the body makes from tryptophan, eating tryptophan-rich foods will boost your melatonin and in turn help you to sleep.

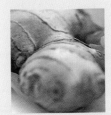 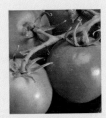 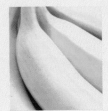

EATING TO COMBAT JET LAG

According to the University of Chicago anti-jet-lag diet, the following schedule will help you when travelling over time zones:

3 DAYS BEFORE FLYING	High protein breakfast and lunch High carbohydrate evening meal
2 DAYS BEFORE FLYING	Approximately 700 calories (fasting)
1 DAY BEFORE FLYING	As 3 days before flying
DAY OF FLYING	As 2 days before flying, with high-protein meal at local breakfast time

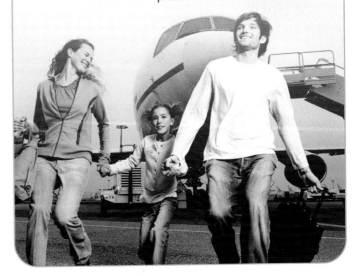

dopamine keeps you active

The neurotransmitter dopamine keeps your brain alert and active. It is involved in thinking and concentration, short-term memory, motivation, emotions including feelings of pleasure, and sexual desire. It also enables you to control and coordinate your movements, and it helps your body to regulate its production of hormones, including the insulin that controls your blood sugar levels.

Dopamine and the closely related noradrenaline (see page 18) are members of a small group of biochemicals called catecholamines, which are produced in brain and nerve cells and in the adrenal glands, a pair of triangular-shaped glands sited on top of the kidneys. The catecholamines that originate in brain and nerve cells act as neurotransmitters, but those that come from the adrenal glands enter the bloodstream and act as hormones. These are chemical messengers that control the functions of the body's organs and tissues.

Making dopamine

Your brain makes the dopamine it needs from the amino acid tyrosine, which it gets from proteins in the food you eat or by making it from another amino acid, phenylalanine. It first uses the enzyme tyrosine hydroxylase to convert the tyrosine into a chemical called L-dopa (or levodopa), then uses another enzyme, L-aromatic amino acid decarboxylase, to convert the L-dopa into dopamine.

So the production of dopamine is similar to that of serotonin—enzymes convert an amino acid into a neurotransmitter. But while eating proteins and other foods rich in the amino acid tryptophan can boost your serotonin levels, eating lots of tyrosine-rich foods won't automatically increase the amount of dopamine in your brain. Your brain makes only as much as it needs, and it only needs to increase dopamine production when there is increased activity in the cells and nerves that use it, as happens when you are under stress.

This means that tyrosine-rich foods don't have much benefit when all is calm and stable, but they can be helpful when the going is tough or stressful. There is some evidence that high doses of tyrosine supplement can improve performance in stressful situations, but it is better to think of tyrosine-rich foods as natural stress busters and perhaps (mild) antidepressants, especially for someone who has become socially withdrawn.

parkinson's disease

This condition is associated with an almost total lack of dopamine in some parts of the brain. Because one of dopamine's functions is to enable the brain to control the body's movements, the lack of dopamine causes symptoms such as muscle tremors, rigidity and difficulty in moving and walking. These symptoms can be greatly reduced, although not entirely eliminated, by taking L-dopa, a synthetic form of the naturally occurring body chemical, which the brain can convert into dopamine.

the chemistry of mood

Too little and too much

Although the brain is good at maintaining its levels of dopamine, sometimes things can go wrong and it produces too little or too much. Some depressed people, for example, may have too little dopamine where it matters, in areas deep within the brain, such as the limbic system, where scientists believe many of the neurochemical processes that mediate mood are located. Such people may find extra tyrosine helpful, together with drugs such as bupropion (Zyban) that act to increase dopamine levels. Bupropion also is used to help people stop smoking. It seems that lack of dopamine is associated with craving, so that boosting its levels with drugs (or tyrosine) can reduce craving.

Problems also can arise if the brain produces too much dopamine, as it is the main neurotransmitter involved in schizophrenia. Of course, schizophrenia is a complicated condition, and many other chemicals are involved as well, but dopamine remains the favoured target of antipsychotic drugs, and there are few, if any, effective drug treatments for schizophrenia that do not in some way block the action of dopamine.

Several dietary interventions can help schizophrenia, and we cover these in more detail later (see page 87). For the time being, we will just mention that animal protein is particularly rich in dopamine, and so a shift towards a vegetarian diet may be advisable for some people with schizophrenia.

good sources of tyrosine

Tyrosine-rich foods include cheese and other dairy products, beer, wine, beans, chicken, liver, fish, sauerkraut, chocolate, bacon, ham, sausage, aubergines, potatoes, spinach and tomatoes.

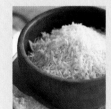 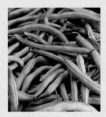 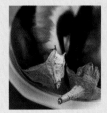

CLINICAL CASEBOOK
THE PLEASURE FACTOR

Enjoyable activities, such as eating, trigger a release of dopamine within the brain that creates feelings of pleasure and satisfaction. The dopamine, like other neurotransmitters, carries signals from one neuron to another, and it triggers pleasure-inducing activity in the receiving neurons by latching onto proteins on their surfaces called dopamine receptors.

Researchers at the Brookhaven National Laboratory on Long Island, New York, have discovered a possible link between dopamine and obesity. Brain scans of obese people showed that they had fewer dopamine receptors than normal, suggesting that those people had to eat more to get the same level of dopamine-induced satisfaction than people with normal numbers of dopamine receptors experience.

noradrenaline to fight or flee?

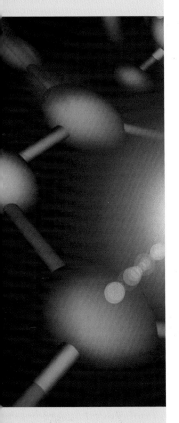

Also known as norepinephrine, noradrenaline is a neurotransmitter produced in your brain and the adrenal glands from dopamine (see page 16). Like dopamine it keeps your brain alert and active and is involved in thinking, concentration and motivation. It also plays a part in moodiness and aggression, the perception of pain, and our responses to stress and danger.

Your brain and adrenal glands use vitamin C and the enzyme dopamine beta-hydroxylase to convert dopamine into noradrenaline, and they can then use another enzyme, called phenylethanolamine-N-methyl transferase, to convert the noradrenaline into the very similar chemical adrenaline (epinephrine).

Both noradrenaline and adrenaline act as neurotransmitters in your brain and nerves, but when released into the bloodstream by the adrenal glands they act as hormones. In their role as hormones, their main effects include increasing your heart-rate and raising your blood pressure when you are excited or frightened.

Highs and lows

The levels of noradrenaline in your brain can have a big effect on your mood. Too much noradrenaline can make you excitable or anxious, while too little can lead to depression.

Some antidepressants that increase the available noradrenaline alone, or increase both noradrenaline and adrenaline, can be more effective than purely serotonin-boosting drugs. These antidepressants make more noradrenaline (or serotonin) available by inhibiting its re-uptake (removal) from the synaptic gap (see page 11) and so increasing the duration of its action. They are especially effective in the more severe or treatment-resistant forms of depression and, because noradrenaline reduces the brain's perception of pain, they can also be effective painkillers. Examples of "noradrenergic" antidepressants are mirtazapine (Remeron, Zispin), venlafaxine (Effexor, Efexor), reboxetine (Edronax), duloxetine (Cymbalta), and milnacipran (Ixel). Apart from reboxetine, these act on the seratonin system, too.

Low levels of available noradrenaline may also play a part in attention deficit and hyperactivity disorders. Low noradrenaline levels make the individual unable to concentrate or focus on one thing at a time and vulnerable to distraction and overstimulation.

Other conditions that involve low noradrenaline levels include Alzheimer's disease, Parkinson's disease, and Korsakov's syndrome (amnesic syndrome). Korsakov's syndrome is a disorder associated with chronic alcoholism and it includes impaired memory and learning ability.

noradrenaline and adrenaline

Noradrenaline, which occurs both in the synapses of brain and nerve cells and in the adrenal glands, functions mainly as a neurotransmitter but is also a hormone. Adrenaline occurs mainly in the adrenal gland, with relatively small amounts in the synapses, and so its role as a hormone is more important than its function as a neurotransmitter.

Noradrenaline and fatigue

We now know that noradrenaline also plays a crucial part in maintaining general alertness, and that fatigue can be due, in part at least, to low levels of noradrenaline.

You can find out if this may apply to you by taking a test dose of no more than 1 gram of the supplement L-tyrosine (available in many health food stores and pharmacies). If you find that your fatigue lifts about 30–60 minutes after this test dose, you may find that increasing the amounts of tyrosine-rich foods in your diet may reduce—or even eliminate—your fatigue. If your noradrenaline levels are normal to begin with, though, taking an L-tyrosine supplement will make little or no difference.

good sources of noradrenaline

Because noradrenaline is made from dopamine, which is made from tyrosine, the same tyrosine-rich foods that promote dopamine production will help to ensure adequate levels of noradrenaline—cheese and other dairy products, beer, wine, beans, chicken, liver, fish, sauerkraut, chocolate, bacon, ham, sausage, aubergines, potatoes, spinach and tomatoes.

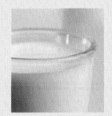 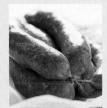 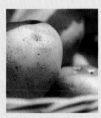

THE FIGHT-OR-FLIGHT RESPONSE

When you are confronted with a sudden and possibly dangerous situation, even something as simple as being startled by a loud noise, your brain and adrenal glands release large amounts of noradrenaline and adrenaline. This "adrenaline rush" is a survival mechanism that prepares you for immediate action.

Your brain produces more noradrenaline so that you become more alert and focus quickly on the source and nature of the threat. Then the nerve endings acting on your heart, blood vessels, lungs and other organs release noradrenaline, and your adrenal glands produce adrenaline, noradrenaline and a range of hormones including cortisol.

In response to this flood of neurotransmitters and hormones, long-term body functions such as digestion are temporarily shut down to divert blood and energy to your brain and muscles; your heart-rate and blood pressure increase; your blood sugar level rises; your bronchial passages open up to allow more air into your lungs; and your perception of pain is dulled. All this is designed to prepare your brain and body for "fight or flight", for confronting the threat or escaping from it.

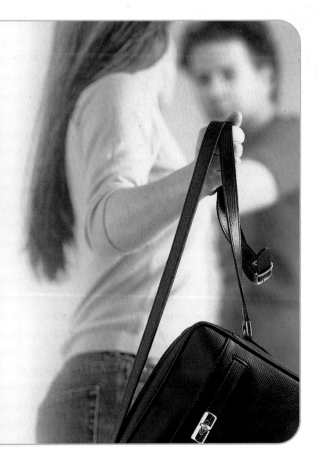

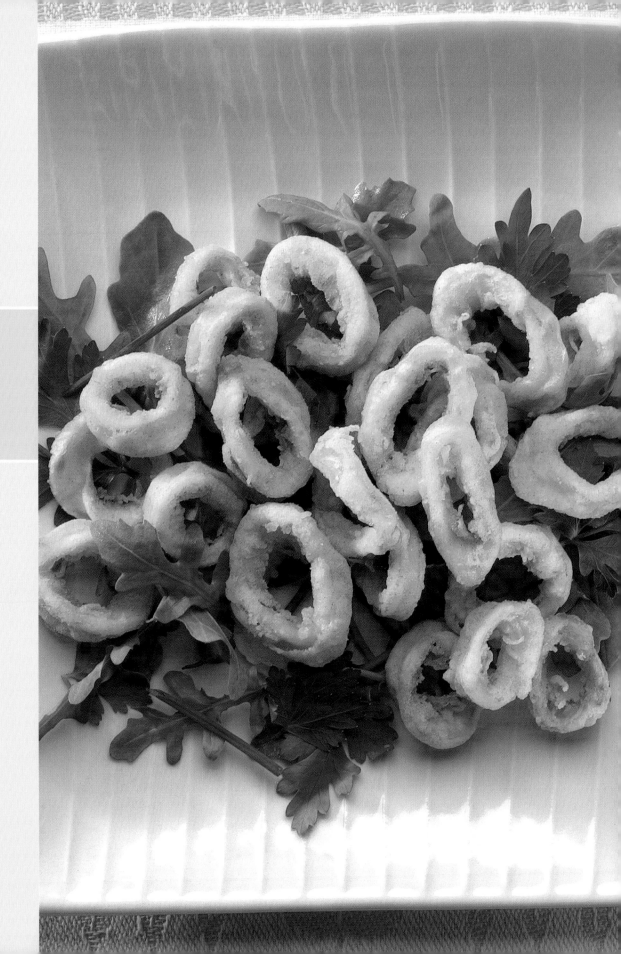

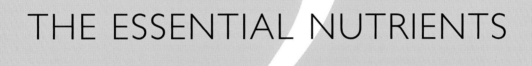

2

THE ESSENTIAL NUTRIENTS

proteins and amino acids

The human body contains more than 10,000 different proteins, which help to build the structure of body cells and tissues such as muscle, skin, bone and hair, as well as the cells of the internal organs, the brain and the nervous system. And specialized types of proteins, called enzymes, control the chemical reactions that enable body and brain cells to function.

Proteins are essential to the maintenance of life, and the World Health Organization has recommended that we get about 10 percent of our total calorie intake from them. This equates to about 35 to 45 grams of protein each day.

Amino acids

All proteins are made from substances called amino acids, and when you eat protein foods your body breaks them down into separate amino acids then reassembles them into the exact types of proteins it needs. It also uses some amino acids as neurotransmitters (see page 10), the chemicals that enable brain and nerve cells to communicate. Glycine, aspartate, and gamma aminobutyric acid (GABA) are important amino acid neurotransmitters, and other major neurotransmitters are made from amino acids. These include serotonin (made from tryptophan) and dopamine (made from tyrosine and phenylalanine).

In total there are some twenty or so amino acids, of which eight—tryptophan, valine, leucine, isoleucine, methionine, phenylalanine, threonine, and lysine—are "essential" amino acids that we cannot make ourselves and therefore must get from our food. Others, such as tyrosine and alanine, are called "nonessential" because they can usually be made by our bodies. A third class of amino acids, the "semi-essential" or "conditionally essential" amino acids, are normally made in the body, but sometimes we need more of them than we can make so we must get them from our food. One of these is glutamine, which is the most common amino acid in the body. Glutamine is made in the muscles and involved in many chemical reactions within the body, especially in the muscles and kidneys, but it is rapidly used up when we are under severe physical stress. Within the brain, glutamine is converted into another amino acid, glutamic acid (glutamate), and then this is converted into the neurotransmitter GABA (see page 11).

Sources of protein

You can get the proteins you need from a wide range of foods—meat, fish, eggs, dairy products, vegetables, cereals, beans, nuts and soya products. Most proteins from meat, fish and eggs are "complete"

taurine for tranquillity

Taurine is an amino acid that is not involved in the making of proteins within the body, but it is present in the brain, eyes, muscles and blood cells. It has a wide range of functions within the body, many of which are not well understood, but it is an antioxidant and also seems extremely important in normal brain development and in aspects of digestion. Taurine is not abundant in plant products, but animal products such as meat, shellfish and cheese (especially cottage cheese) are rich in it. Because taurine has a calming effect on the brain, these are excellent foods to counter anxiety.

THE GOODNESS OF GLUTAMINE

Glutamine is supposed to improve your mood, and glutamine supplements and glutamine-rich foods are claimed to help reduce cravings for drugs, especially alcohol. Some studies conclude that glutamine is helpful in these conditions while others say that it makes no difference whatsoever, but glutamine supplements are in general not harmful, so they may be worth trying despite the conflicting evidence.

proteins because they contain all the essential amino acids. But proteins from other sources (except soya) tend to lack one or more of the essential amino acids, so if you are a vegetarian you should get your protein from soya or from a good mix of foods, including vegetables, beans, lentils and nuts, to make sure you get all the amino acids your body needs.

Although meat and fish are excellent sources of protein, most red meat contains a lot of fat, so eating too much of it can be unhealthy in the long term. Meats such as poultry (especially with the skin removed) and venison are less fatty, so they are better sources of protein than many red meats.

The joy of soya

Soya products, including tofu, soya flour and dried soya beans, contain more protein, weight-for-weight, than meat or other animal products. Among plant proteins, the soya bean is the only one to contain all the eight essential amino acids—including lysine, an amino acid that is uncommon in most plant proteins.

Soya products are also rich in phospholipids, especially phosphatidyl choline (see page 26), which is thought to be a helpful booster for brain function in general and memory function in particular. And because there are very few saturated fats and no cholesterol in soya products, tofu is one of those rare high-protein foods that is low in calories and free of cholesterol.

Although the relationship between cholesterol in food and artery-clogging cholesterol in the blood is controversial (and is probably not a very close relationship), soya products including tofu are widely recommended protein sources for people with heart disease. This is because as well as containing no cholesterol, they can reduce the levels of harmful cholesterol in the bloodstream. They are also excellent sources of calcium, iron, phosphorus, B-group vitamins, choline, and vitamin E.

did you know?

Although eating soya products is a healthy way to get the proteins you need, it is probably unwise to eat too much of them. This is because soya contains substances called isoflavones, which have effects similar to those of the hormone oestrogen. Some studies suggest that a diet high in isoflavones may reduce the risk of breast cancer, but others indicate that it may increase this risk. Because of this contradictory evidence, the American Cancer Society has concluded that people who have had breast cancer, or who are at high risk of the disease, should eat only moderate amounts of soya products.

essential fats the omega factor

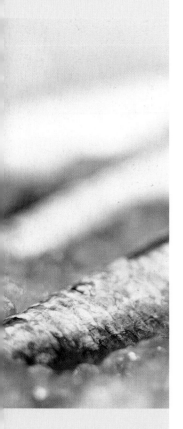

If you were asked to list the parts of your body that contain a lot of fat, you probably wouldn't include your brain, but fatty substances make up more than sixty percent of your brain tissue. These fatty substances help form the structures of the brain cells, and may help the cells to communicate effectively.

Structural v storage

The fat content of your brain is called structural fat, which is very different to the storage fat that your body uses as an energy reserve to keep it going when food is in short supply. Storage fat is the fat that accumulates around your waist and hips when you become overweight. In the brain, structural fat combines with proteins and other materials to form the structures of the cells, including their outer membranes and the myelin sheaths of the axons.

Fats are formed when substances called fatty acids combine with glycerol (glycerine), a type of alcohol. Fatty acids can be either saturated or unsaturated, and the most important for the brain's structure and function are the omega 3 and omega 6 groups of unsaturated fatty acids.

We humans (in common with all other animals with backbones) are unable to produce omega 3 and omega 6 fatty acids ourselves, so we must get them from the foods we eat.

Research indicates that for good physical health and brain function, we need roughly equal amounts of omega 3 and omega 6 fatty acids in our diet. The current Western diet typically contains plenty of omega 6 but comparatively little omega 3. This is in contrast to the Japanese diet, in which the amounts of omega 3 and omega 6 are nearly equal.

The most important omega 3 fatty acids are docosahexanoic acid (DHA), eicosapentanoic acid (EPA), and alpha-linolenic acid (ALA). DHA and EPA are known as long-chain omega 3 fatty acids and are found mainly in fish oil and coldwater oily fish, such as anchovies, mackerel and bonito. ALA is mainly derived from plants, such as flaxseed (linseed) and others.

The Japanese diet is rich in omega 3 fatty acids because it includes a lot of fish, and the Western diet is poor in omega 3 because fish is not such an important part of it. Omega 6 fatty acids include linoleic acid (LA) and arachidonic acid (AA), which come mainly from vegetable oils and are widespread in Western diets.

Mood improvers

Increased levels of omega 3 fatty acids appear to benefit people with mood disorders. It is not known precisely how they do this, but there is mounting

trans fatty acids

These are formed from the partial breakdown of vegetable and fish oils. For food manufacturers, they help to stabilize butter substitutes and are widely used in shortening and deep-frying. It seems that if you consume trans fatty acids in large amounts you are likely to increase your "bad" (LDL) cholesterol and reduce your "good" (HDL) cholesterol. Not all trans fatty acids are the same, and the debate is complex, but we advise you to cut down your use of them. There is increasing pressure on snack manufacturers to cut their use of trans fatty acids.

evidence that they have similar effects to the so-called "mood stabilizer" drugs such as lithium. And in several small-scale studies, high doses of omega 3 fatty acids (almost 10 grams per day) produced a response that was better than with an inactive placebo (olive oil) in people who had recently been manic.

There also is growing evidence that omega 3 fatty acids can be helpful in depression, particularly in the depression that women can suffer after giving birth (postnatal depression). A developing foetus and the newborn baby need large amounts of omega 3 fatty acids in order to develop, and their only sources for this are first the placenta and then breast milk. The baby is able to "drain" omega 3 fatty acids from its mother, so she is more

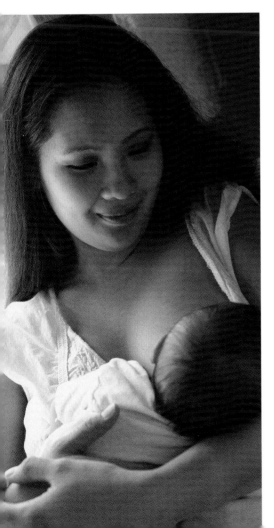

Good sources of essential fats

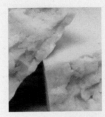 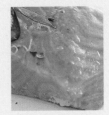 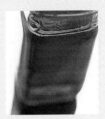

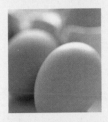

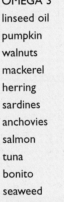

OMEGA 3	OMEGA 6
linseed oil	corn oil
pumpkin	sunflower oil
walnuts	sesame oil
mackerel	meat
herring	milk
sardines	cheese
anchovies	eggs
salmon	squid
tuna	
bonito	
seaweed	
eggs	

likely to suffer lower omega 3 levels unless these are supplemented in the diet. It appears that depletion of brain and body omega 3 fatty acids leads to a greater risk of becoming depressed, but we don't yet know why.

There have been reports that depression is lower in countries such as Japan, where fish figures strongly in the diet. On the other hand, recent population studies in Japan indicate that depression is commoner there than previously thought, and the suicide rate in Japan is higher than that in the West.

Phospholipids
Among the most important structural fats in the body and brain are phospholipids,

good sources of phospholipids

FOOD
Eggs are rich in phospholipids, and although they are also high in cholesterol, most research shows that eating eggs makes no difference on the cholesterol level in your blood.
Sardines and nuts are also good sources.

SUPPLEMENTS
Lecithin, generally found as a supplement in granule or capsule form, is another important source of phospholipids. An adequate supplement would be a tablespoonful of lecithin, sprinkled on cereal or salad.

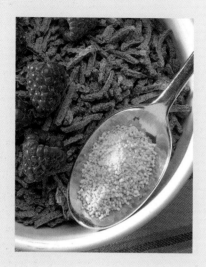

which include both saturated and unsaturated fatty acids combined with phosphorus. The outer membranes of most cells, including brain cells, are made of double layers of phospholipids interspersed with proteins, and the myelin sheaths of axons are formed from them. The two main varieties of phospholipids are phosphatidyl choline and phosphatidyl serine.

The body is able to make its own phospholipids, but there is some evidence that adding extra phospholipids to the diet can improve overall brain function including memory and thinking abilities.

Fatty acids and the fats that they make are crucial to brain function, memory and learning capability, as well as improving mood in general.

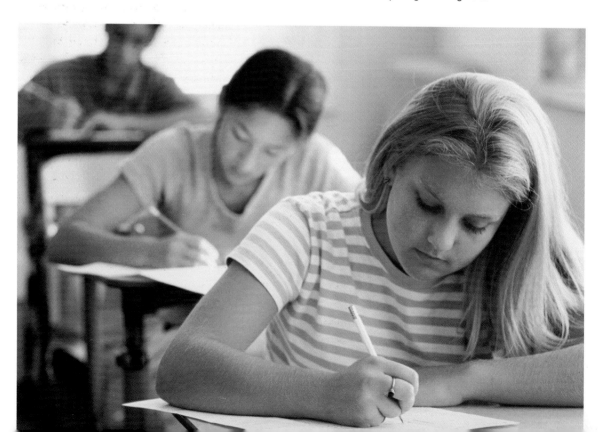

glucose for power

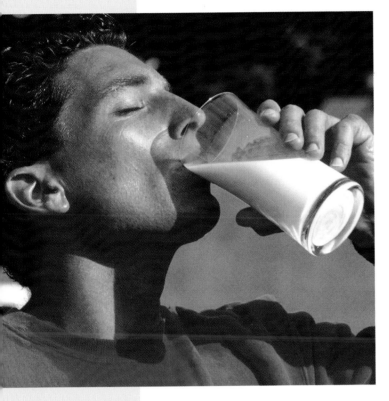

A type of sugar, glucose, is perhaps the most important chemical of all because without it the brain simply cannot function—it needs glucose to produce the energy that powers it. Few foods contain glucose itself, so the body makes most of its glucose from the carbohydrates (sugars and starches) and fats that are widely available in foods.

Glucose is extracted from food by the digestive system and carried around the body in the bloodstream, and the levels of glucose in the blood (the "blood sugar levels") are controlled by a complex group of chemicals of which insulin, produced by the pancreas, is perhaps the best known. Insulin also controls the passage of glucose into cells. Without it, wide and rapid fluctuations of glucose

level could impair the performance of the brain and, in extreme cases, be actively harmful to some of the brain cells.

The insulin system is extremely efficient, although it does not react instantaneously to fluctuations in glucose levels, and low blood glucose can have a noticeable impact on your mood. For example, you may feel irritable and your attention may flag as the previous meal time recedes and your blood glucose levels fall.

Getting a rapid "hit" of glucose by eating chocolate or ice cream can temporarily lift your mood, but the whole system works best if the supply of glucose—and thus of the energy it provides—is more controlled. This is where choice of food becomes important, because not all sources of glucose are the same. Refined sugars, honey and syrups, cause a rapid increase in glucose levels. Fruit sugar (fructose) results in slightly slower but longer-lasting increases, and the glucose in carbohydrate foods such as bread or pasta is released even more slowly.

Simple and complex carbohydrates

The sugars and starches from which our bodies get most of their energy-providing glucose are carbohydrates, substances made up of atoms of carbon, hydrogen, and oxygen. The most basic carbohydrates are the simple sugars such as glucose and fructose (fruit sugar), which can combine to form more complex sugars such as sucrose (cane or beet sugar). Starches consist of molecules of glucose linked together in long chains, and plants make them as a convenient way of storing glucose as an energy reserve.

The glycaemic index

The way in which a food affects the glucose levels in your bloodstream is measured by its glycaemic index (GI). The GI of a food compares the increase in your blood glucose levels after you eat a standard amount of it with how much they increase if you eat a standard amount of pure glucose. So the glycaemic index of pure glucose is, by definition, 100, but oatmeal increases your blood glucose levels by half the amount that pure glucose does, so its GI is 50, and that of peanuts is less than 20. While it is possible for a food to have a GI of greater than 100 (as jasmine rice does, for example), most foods have a lower GI than that of pure glucose. As far as the brain is concerned, the lower the glycaemic index, the more controlled the glucose levels will be.

Researchers have measured the glycaemic indexes of most common foods. Usually, as in this book, a low glycaemic index is defined as a GI of less than 50, and anything higher is defined as a high GI. But you might also see a high GI classified as one that is greater than 70 and a low GI as less than 55, with GIs in between these referred to as medium. Another complication is that some indexes take white bread as the reference food, and give it a GI of 100. On these indexes, pure glucose has a GI of 140.

Whether you are diabetic or not, you can use the glycaemic index to help plan healthy meals that will give a controlled, sustained release of energy.

However, it is unwise to be obsessional about the precise glycaemic index of the food you eat. Instead, just try some simple changes in your eating habits that will help you to reduce the overall GI of your diet and avoid peaks and troughs in your blood glucose levels. Opt for breakfast cereals based on wheat, bran, and oats; for breads made with whole grains; for spaghetti, rice or buckwheat instead of potatoes; and for vinaigrette salad dressing instead of a creamy or cheese-based dressing. Increasing the number of portions of fruit and vegetables you eat each day, and reducing the amount of sugary food you eat, will also help.

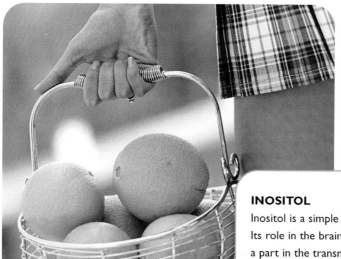

INOSITOL

Inositol is a simple carbohydrate chemically related to glucose. Its role in the brain is not entirely clear but it probably plays a part in the transmission of messages between and within neurons, and there is some evidence that inositol supplements can help relieve depression, panic, obsessions, and bulimia. It can be found in dried peas and beans, lentils, soya flour, eggs, fish, liver, citrus fruits and nuts.

high-glycaemic-index foods (GI greater than 50)

glucose	cornflakes	potato crisps	rice cakes
honey	wholemeal bread	bagels	biscuits
refined sugar	waffles	pumpkin	sweets
muesli	crispbread	melon	lemonades
whole-wheat cereals	parsnips	pineapple	colas
white bread	potatoes	bananas	
French bread	French fries	rice	

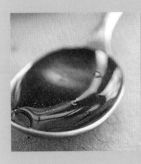 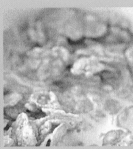 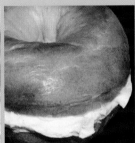 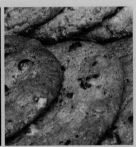

low-glycaemic-index foods (GI less than 50)

fructose	cherries	pasta	peas
grapes	fruit juice	whole-grain bread	most beans (including
oranges	milk	oats	baked beans)
apples	yoghurt	bran	
pears	nuts	carrots	

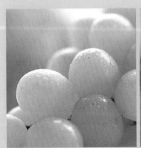 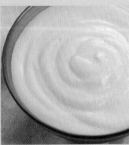 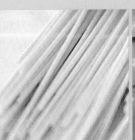 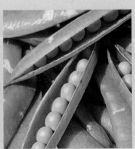

sources of nutrients

The essential principle of healthy eating is maintaining a balanced diet, one that contains all the essential nutrients including proteins, carbohydrates, fats, fibre, vitamins and minerals. The nutrients listed here are those known to be beneficial to your mental health, and by ensuring that your normal diet includes foods that contain them, you will avoid deficiencies that could have a negative effect on your mental health.

the food pyramid

The Food Pyramid, devised by the US Department of Agriculture (USDA), is a visual image that illustrates how much of each type of food you should eat each day to achieve a healthy diet. The pyramid has four levels, with bread, grains and cereals making up the large base. Vegetables and fruits make up the next level, followed by meat and milk products as the third level and fats, oils and sweets making up the small tip of the pyramid.

Build up your daily diet in the same way. Eat lots of bread, cereals, rice and pasta, plus plenty of vegetables and fruits, two or three servings each of meat and milk products, and sparing amounts of additional fats, oils and sweeteners.

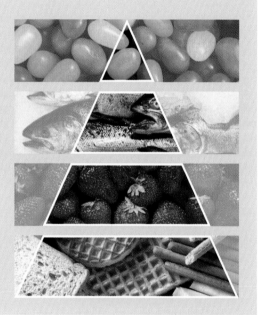

b-group vitamins

VITAMIN B_1 (thiamin)	VITAMIN B_3 (niacin)	VITAMIN B_6 (pyridoxal)	VITAMIN B_{12} (cobalamin)	FOLIC ACID (folate)
wheatgerm	whole grains	whole grains	milk	leafy vegetables
whole grains	dried beans	lean meat	cheese	dried beans
dried beans	fish	fish	eggs	poultry
seafood	poultry	poultry	fish	fortified cereals
		potatoes	poultry	oranges
			lean beef	nuts

minerals and trace elements

CALCIUM

Swiss cheese
Cheddar cheese
almonds
brewer's yeast
pumpkin seeds
beans

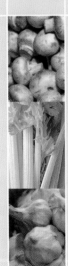

CHROMIUM

Swiss cheese
brewer's yeast
wholemeal bread
potatoes
wheatgerm
green peppers
eggs
chicken
apples
lamb
oysters

IRON

pumpkin seeds
sesame seeds
almonds
cashew nuts
brazil nuts
walnuts
raisins
dates
prunes
pork
beans
parsley

MAGNESIUM

wheatgerm
brewer's yeast
buckwheat flour
almonds
Brazil nuts
cashew nuts
peanuts
beans

MANGANESE

watercress
okra
pineapple
blackberries
raspberries

POTASSIUM

watercress
endive
cabbage
celery
mushrooms
bananas
pumpkin
molasses
garlic
raisins
peas
crab

SELENIUM

Brazil nuts
tuna
oysters
mushrooms
herring

ZINC

Brazil nuts
almonds
oysters
shrimp
haddock
eggs
oats
ginger root
lamb

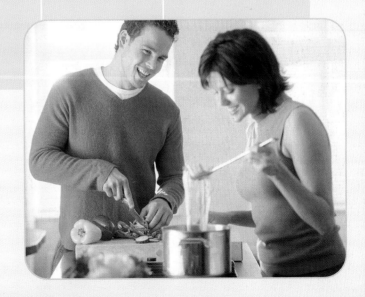

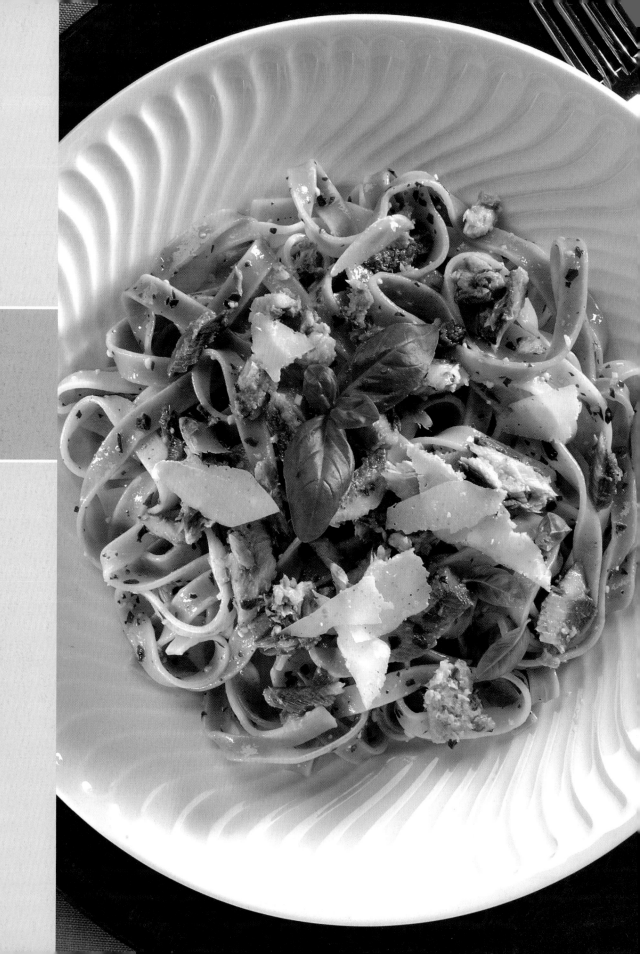

3

WHAT'S THE RIGHT AMOUNT?

eating and good health

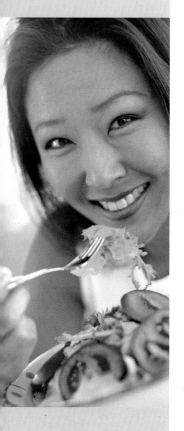

The idea of what makes up a wholesome, balanced diet has evolved over the years as nutritionists have learned more about the nutrients that keep body and brain healthy, and calculated how much of them we need each day.

Eating the right foods will do much to optimize your mental health, and help you to develop a positive outlook on life. The first step is to ensure that the foods you eat give you the nutrients you need for good physical health, and the system of five major food groups (see box, right) provides simple guidelines for this. Using the food groups system as the framework of your diet, you can choose foods that not only fit in with its recommendations but also are of benefit to your brain.

Components of a healthy diet

The five major food groups are bread, grains and cereals; vegetables; fruits; meat, dried beans, nuts and eggs; and dairy products, and if you eat at least the minimum number of servings from each of the groups each day, you will have a balanced diet (see box, right). The fats, oils and sweeteners (such as butter, salad dressings and sugar) that are added to foods make up a sixth, minor, group. You should use these very sparingly, if at all. The food groups system suggests a range of servings for most of the groups, enabling you to choose the numbers of servings that will match your specific daily calorie requirements. What these are will depend on various factors, discussed in detail in the following pages. With the help of these guidelines you can find the amounts and proportions of different foods that you need for good overall health.

Boosting your "happiness" quotient

In terms of brain health and happiness, not all foods are equal. The tables on pages 29–31 set out the items that will do the most to help nourish your brain. Opting for turkey or fish instead of red meat, for example, will provide you with more tryptophan, which will boost your serotonin levels. And if you choose an oily fish such as tuna or salmon instead of cod or sole, you will also get more of the essential omega 3 fatty acids that help your brain cells to function properly.

Are recommended amounts suitable for you?

The science underlying the food groups is based on more than fifty years of research into the nutrients we need for good health. We need enough of each one to avoid the effects of deficiency, but not so much of it that it causes us harm. For example, we need enough iron in our diets to prevent anaemia, but too much of it causes liver damage.

Until recently, the measures of how much of each nutrient we need were the Recommended Dietary Allowances (RDAs). The RDAs are the minimum amounts of a nutrient—whether a macronutrient (such as protein or carbohydrate) or a micronutrient (a vitamin or mineral)—that different groups of people need in their diets.

Today, nutritionists use Dietary Reference Intakes (DRIs) to define our nutrient needs. Unlike RDAs, which just set out our minimum requirements, DRIs set their sights higher because they are designed to aid the planning and evaluation of diets for healthy people. RDAs and DRIs

food groups and daily servings

FOOD GROUP	SERVINGS		TYPICAL SERVING SIZES
bread, grains and cereals	6 to 11		one slice bread 25g (1oz) cereal 100g (3½oz) cooked grain, rice or pasta
vegetables	3 to 5		75g (2¾oz) raw leafy vegetables 40g (1½oz) non-leafy vegetables, cooked or raw 175ml (6fl oz) vegetable juice
fruits	2 to 4		one medium-size fruit, such as an apple 125g (4½oz) chopped fresh, cooked or canned fruit 40g (1½oz) dried fruit 175ml (6fl oz) fruit juice
meat, dried beans, nuts, eggs	2 to 3		85g (3oz) lean meat 85g (3oz) fish 85g (3oz) poultry 35g (1¼oz) nuts 2 tablespoons peanut butter 55g (2oz) cooked dried beans one egg
dairy products	2 to 3		250ml (9fl oz) milk or yoghurt 42g (1½oz) natural cheese 55g (2oz) processed cheese
fats, oils and sweeteners	use sparingly		

are generally well accepted internationally. However, neither goes beyond telling you what makes up a healthy, nutritious diet. They tell you nothing about how nutrients can be used as treatment when things go wrong, or how much more of a particular nutrient you might need to maintain an "extraordinary" lifestyle. They don't take food production into account, either. Each new food scandal throws more light into the murkier areas of what happens to our food before it's brought to the table, such as over-fertilized vegetables, or cattle and poultry fed on antibiotics. Can we trust what we eat? Dietitians suggest that everyone should take multivitamin supplements. There's not a great deal of hard evidence that you should follow this advice. But a great many of us do.

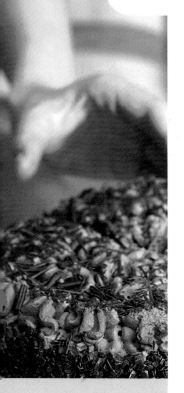

the effects of a bad diet

Your brain and body are linked in complex and subtle ways, so it is not surprising that there are many links between mental and physical health. Because of these links, a bad diet can cause both physical and mental health problems, and psychological disorders can lead to a number of unhealthy physical conditions. For example, psychological disorders underpin eating disorders such as anorexia, and may often contribute to the development of obesity.

The overeating that causes obesity can sometimes be triggered by stress, and can both cause and result from poor self-image and low self-esteem. Overeating and obesity also can lead to many physical health problems, from a lack of energy to high blood pressure and heart disease, and may contribute to the onset of diabetes.

Diabetes

An extremely common disorder—around 200 million people worldwide suffer from diabetes, and the numbers are rising rapidly. When someone has diabetes, his

SUGARY BEER
Many alcoholic drinks, especially beer, have large amounts of sugars. These are chiefly in the form of maltose, which consists of two glucose molecules linked together, so there is a lot of glucose in a glass of beer. This may account for the weight gain in regular beer drinkers.

or her body is unable to control its levels of blood sugar, which become consistently high (hyperglycaemia) but may fluctuate and become too low (hypoglycaemia). The levels of sugar in the blood normally are controlled by the hormone insulin, which is produced in the pancreas.

There are two main types of diabetes, type I and type II. People with type I diabetes need to inject themselves with extra insulin to control the condition, while those with type II diabetes do not. In type I diabetes, one of the main problems is that the body produces too little insulin. In type II diabetes, the problem is not necessarily that there is too little insulin (although this may be the case), but that the cells and tissues on which insulin normally acts are relatively insensitive to its effects.

Genetics can play an important part in your risk of developing diabetes. There are some comparatively rare genetic conditions that can cause diabetes in a few families, and people from some ethnic backgrounds, such as Africans, Afro-Caribbeans, African-Americans, and people from some parts of Asia, are

healthy weight loss

This is not a weight loss diet book, although our recipes are healthy and not especially fattening. However, there are simple principles that govern healthy weight loss. Firstly, yo-yo or starvation dieting is at best unsuccessful in the long run, and at worst dangerous. Aim to lose no more than 450g (1lb) per week. Diets high in protein may help you lose weight, but most nutritionists advocate a balance between fat and fibre, carbohydrate and protein. In general, pick low GI foods (see page 29) with a lower density (energy by weight), such as fruit and vegetables, over high density or processed foods, and reduce your salt intake.

particularly vulnerable to the condition. However, several risk factors are important in the development of diabetes, especially of the more common type II. Chief among these is obesity, one of the leading causes of type II diabetes.

Diet and diabetes

A combination of family history, membership of a higher-risk ethnic group, lack of exercise, and a high-fat, high-sugar diet, is much more likely to lead to obesity and diabetes than a normal balanced diet, especially one that includes plenty of fruit and vegetables.

Although the levels of insulin in your bloodstream are controlled by many factors, the amount of sugar in your blood is the most important. After a meal, the sugar in your blood increases. Then the levels of insulin rise to deal with the increased sugar, and the sugar level falls again. Some researchers have suggested, admittedly mainly from experimental rather than clinical studies, that long-term intake of sugar can increase the level of insulin demand so much that the pancreas can no longer cope and diabetes follows.

Eating sugar in itself does not cause diabetes, but everyone should try to limit the amount of sugar he or she eats, and take account of the speeds at which different foods release their sugar content into the bloodstream. The glycaemic index of foods (see page 28) is an important way of comparing the sugar release from different foods—you should eat high-glycaemic-index foods more sparingly, especially if you have diabetes.

You also should beware of the hidden sugar content of many processed foods. Economy brands, in particular, are likely to contain added sugar, but you should always read labels carefully even if the box promises "no added sugar".

can chromium help?

Chromium helps the body to use insulin more effectively, so if you have type II diabetes you may benefit from increasing the amount of chromium in your diet. You can do this by taking chromium supplements, or by eating foods that are rich in chromium, such as broccoli and other greens, tomatoes, raw onions and poultry, especially turkey. Chromium seems to be well-tolerated by the body, although very high doses may affect the kidneys.

Children seem especially susceptible to changes in glucose levels, but it may depend on their personalities. Active children show increased blood glucose levels when stressed, compared with calmer children.

Psychiatric disorders, especially depression, don't cause diabetes but can make the blood sugar more difficult to control, but control is improved if the depression is treated, and the depression seems to improve if the blood sugar is better controlled.

There has recently been an enormous increase in the numbers of children suffering from diabetes. This is being blamed on diets with a surfeit of sweet foods.

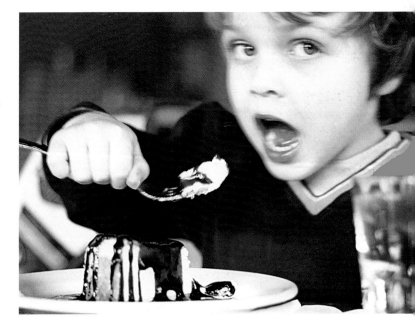

your changing needs

Our brains need proper feeding throughout life, from conception onward. During infancy and childhood, a healthy diet helps your brain to grow, and sets up the trillions of internal connections that link your cells and enable them to function. In adulthood, it supplies the nutrients that your brain needs both to keep it working properly, and to combat wear and tear and the inevitable effects of the ageing process.

The basic framework of a healthy diet (see page 34) applies from childhood through to old age—lots of grains, cereals, vegetables and fruits, plus small helpings of meat and dairy products and sparing amounts of fats, sweeteners and oils. A diet like this will give you all the nutrients you need for optimum physical and mental health, provided you fine-tune it to allow for the way the body's needs change throughout life.

Pregnancy—eating for two

When a woman is pregnant, she needs extra nutrients to protect both her own health and that of her developing baby. So during pregnancy your appetite will increase, but your calorie consumption needs to be kept in check. You should ask your doctor to advise you on your recommended calorie intake, but in general a normal-weight woman should keep her calorie consumption at its usual level for the first three months of pregnancy and increase it by 300 calories (1255 kilojoules) a day for the last six months. Eat extra fruit and vegetables to satisfy your increased hunger, and carbohydrates, proteins and yoghurt to provide the extra calories.

But "eating for two" does not mean simply eating more. As well as extra calories, you need more of certain vitamins and minerals while you are pregnant, and you also need to take extra precautions with your food. However, it's wise to take supplements because your normal diet (especially if you are often too nauseated to eat) probably won't supply enough folic acid, vitamins, iron and calcium for both you and your baby.

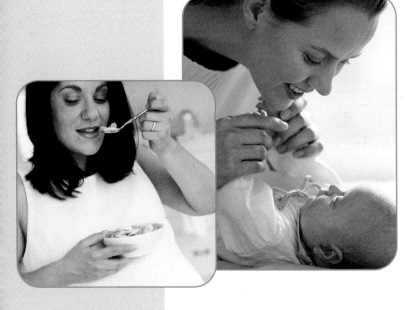

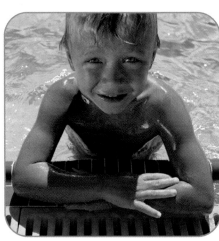

Supplements

Folic acid is essential for the normal development of your baby's nervous system. You also should take folic acid supplements (400 micrograms per day) during the first few weeks of pregnancy. Eat plenty of foods rich in folic acid, such as enriched bread, chicken liver (in small quantities—large amounts contain too much vitamin A, which can cause birth defects), leafy green vegetables, lentils, asparagus, eggs and salmon.

It's easy to become deficient in iron when you are pregnant. Unless your blood haemoglobin level is low, most doctors will not recommend treatment with iron supplements because they can provide too much iron (see page 90), but a daily multivitamin supplement containing iron will do no harm. Red meat is an excellent dietary source of iron, but too much of this is undesirable so seeds and nuts, also rich sources of iron, are better options.

Care with foods

Meat, poultry, eggs, fish and seafood should be cooked thoroughly to destroy any harmful bacteria. Avoid unwashed vegetables and salads, and unpasteurized milk or milk products, especially soft, blue-veined, or mould-ripened cheeses, fresh pâtés, or unheated cooked-chilled meals that cannot be reheated safely. Make sure any reheated food is piping hot, don't refreeze food once it has been defrosted, and store raw and cooked foods separately.

Feeding your new baby

Breast milk is the perfect food for infants because it contains all the essential nutrients that a baby needs, plus antibodies that boost his or her immune system and offer protection from infections. Infant formula, whether milk-based or soya-based, also provides all the essential nutrients but it lacks protective antibodies.

Although breastfeeding is usually better for your baby than formula feeding, it is important not to feel guilty if breastfeeding is not for you because it is too difficult or painful. But if you are able to breastfeed for a short while before switching to formula—even for

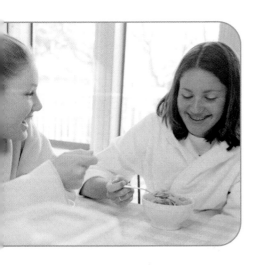

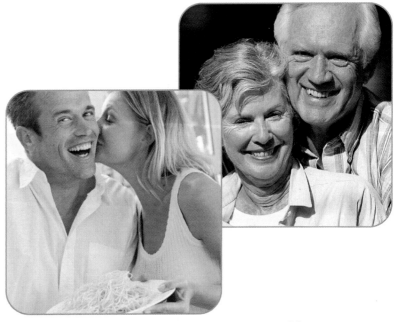

A HEALTHY LIFESTYLE

To maximize the physical and mental benefits of eating a healthy diet, you need to combine it with a healthy lifestyle, for example by limiting your alcohol consumption, quitting smoking, and avoiding other recreational drugs. You should also try to get your weight down (or perhaps up) to roughly what is considered normal for someone of your height, build and gender, and then tailor your daily energy (calorie) intake to a level that keeps you at that weight.

Keeping yourself active is another important part of a healthy lifestyle. Regular moderate exercise—such as 30 minutes of brisk walking or cycling—burns up excess calories, strengthens your heart and lungs, and improves your circulatory system, making it better able to deliver oxygen and nutrients to your muscles and brain and carry away waste products and toxins. It also strengthens your muscles, bones and joints, improves the condition of your skin, and stimulates the release of endorphins, stress-relieving brain chemicals that create feelings of pleasure and happiness.

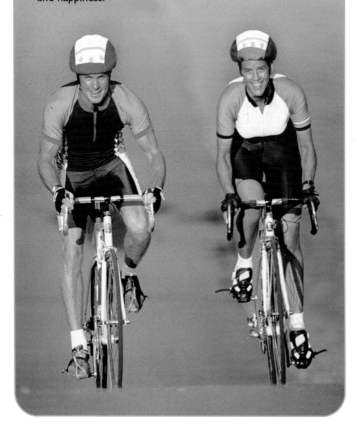

just the first three weeks—your baby will get a good supply of antibodies. If you do elect for formula feeding, we cannot stress too highly that the instructions for using the formula should be followed to the letter, with careful attention to hygiene.

Whether you are breastfeeding or bottlefeeding your new baby, remember your own dietary needs and continue to eat a healthy, balanced diet. If you are breastfeeding, remember to drink plenty of fluids, which will help you to make breastmilk. While you are breastfeeding, you will need more energy and you should increase your daily calorie intake to about 200 calories (840 kilojoules) more than it was when you were pregnant. If you are bottlefeeding your baby, or have stopped breastfeeding, you won't need the extra energy so you should cut your daily calorie intake to about 300 calories (1255 kilojoules) less than when you were pregnant.

The growing child

Boys and girls have roughly the same nutritional needs, although boys tend to need more calories from the age of about eight until the age of 12, and girls tend to need more protein as they approach puberty. Both need roughly the same amounts of vitamins A, B and C as an adult does, but more iron and more calcium (of which there is more in semi-skimmed than in full-fat milk).

Breakfast is an important meal for children, and research shows that

DAILY CALORIE REQUIREMENTS	
MEN	WOMEN
2500	2000

children who have breakfast (especially foods with a low to medium glycaemic index, see page 29) perform better at their schoolwork and are better behaved. Having a good breakfast also reduces the temptation to snack on sugary and fatty foods during the day.

Sweet foods and the colorants they often contain also have been implicated in childhood behavioural problems (see page 78). Similarly, too much caffeine or other stimulants can make your children overactive, so encourage them to drink fruit juice or water rather than caffeine-rich coffee, tea and cola drinks.

The teen years

Good nutrition is vital in the teenage years because during this time we gain up to half our adult weight, half our adult bone mass, and a fifth of our adult height. Unfortunately, this is also the period when children may be eating least well— less parental supervision, plus money to spend on fast foods, snacks and sugary drinks—and are more resistant to instruction in good eating.

This opportunity to eat badly means that in most developed countries there are significant problems of teenage under-nutrition, stunted growth and obesity, coupled with deficiencies in iron, calcium, iodine and vitamins including folic acid. A balanced diet for adolescents should include plenty of foods rich in these substances.

Entering the adult years

By the time you reach your twenties your body and brain are fully developed. Physical growth has stopped and if, like most people, you gradually become less physically active you will need to cut down on calorie-rich foods to keep your weight under control. Try to shed any bad

did you know?

Some research has indicated that high doses of antioxidants—substances that mop up cell-damaging chemicals called free radicals—may help to slow the ageing process. Common antioxidants include vitamins A, C and E (found in many foods, especially fruit and vegetables) and substances called flavonoids, found in some red wines (especially Merlot). Although the evidence that antioxidants really help is often contradictory and hard to interpret, some people probably benefit from them and moderate doses seem to cause little or no harm.

eating habits you developed as a teenager, and make eating a properly varied diet one of your priorities in life: without good physical and mental health, everything else you do will be diminished.

The older adult

As you pass through middle age you may need to modify your diet, firstly to help you cope better with the effects of menopause or viropause (see page 42) and then to counteract the effects of ageing. For a healthy diet in later life, cut down on artery-clogging saturated fats (found in meat and dairy products) and eat oily fish at least twice a week to help your brain function properly and keep your joints supple. Eat plenty of foods rich in vitamins, iron and dietary fibre, such as fruit, vegetables, nuts and seeds, and cereals, and cut down on salty or smoked foods as they may increase your blood pressure and with it your risk of suffering a stroke. You should also limit your intake of sugary foods, because these contribute to obesity and that may lead to diabetes.

around the time of the menopause

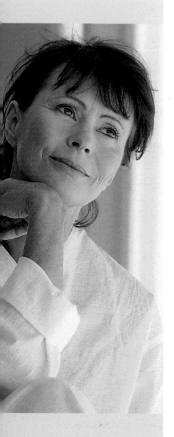

During menopause, the amount of oestrogen and many other hormones circulating in your body drops significantly, and this can leave you vulnerable to a range of physical, psychological and emotional changes including fatigue, insomnia, irritability, anxiety, depression and memory problems, which can undermine your happiness. Many of the these effects are easier to manage if you eat the right foods and adopt a healthy lifestyle.

Some of the changes experienced during this time, such as insomnia caused by hot flushes interrupting your sleep, are directly attributable to the menopause, but others (memory problems, for instance) may just be part of the normal ageing process.

You should be careful to eat plenty of fruit and vegetables, especially oranges, broccoli, spinach, marrow and carrots, to ensure a good supply of important nutrients including vitamins A and D and folic acid, and limit the calories in your diet that come from fat to no more than 30 percent of your daily total.

Phyto- or plant-based oestrogens
The drop in oestrogen levels appears to be at least partly responsible for many unwelcome side effects of menopause. It has been suggested that low oestrogen levels reduce the production of serotonin, possibly leading to moodiness and even depression, and lack of oestrogen may also contribute to hot flushes, fatigue, irritability, insomnia, poor concentration, osteoporosis (loss of bone mass), and even weight gain. Hormone replacement therapy (HRT), which boosts the levels of oestrogen in

your body, will help to combat these problems. But if HRT is not suitable for you (whether for medical reasons or because you are, quite reasonably, unsure about its long-term effects) you might want to try increasing your oestrogen levels by adding extra phyto-oestrogens (plant oestrogens) to your diet. Good sources of phyto-oestrogens include soya beans and soya proteins (such as tofu and soya milk), beans, peas, lentils, fruit, pumpkin seeds and flaxseeds (linseeds).

The effects of adding extra phyto-oestrogens to your diet are very mild compared to the effects of HRT, although phyto-oestrogens appear to reduce the severity and frequency of hot flushes and their consequences, such as insomnia leading to fatigue and irritability. However, phyto-oestrogens do reduce harmful cholesterol in your bloodstream, which cuts your risk of high blood pressure and heart problems in later life, and they also help your bones to absorb more calcium, which makes you less vulnerable to osteoporosis.

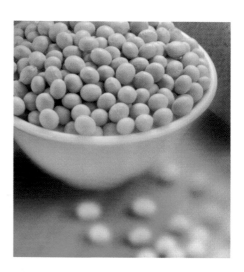

Other useful nutrients

Most authorities agree that pre- and peri-menopausal women need around 1000mg of calcium per day, and after menopause, if you are taking hormone replacement therapy (HRT), you should continue to take about 1000mg per day. If you are not on HRT, you need around 1500mg. Calcium-rich foods include milk and other dairy products, nuts, oysters, sardines (including the bones, if you can stomach them) and canned salmon, as well as spinach, broccoli and other dark-green leafy vegetables.

Vitamin D also is important because it helps your body to utilize calcium, and good sources of vitamin D include milk, eggs, salmon and other oily fish, and fish oils. Sunlight helps your body to synthesize vitamin D from 7-dehydro-cholesterol, a substance present in your skin, so you should increase your vitamin D intake during the winter months when there is less sunlight. You also can take Vitamin D supplements, but seek the advice of your doctor before doing so because high doses of vitamin D cause kidney damage, including painful stones. Recent research has suggested that elderly people taking 800mg of vitamin D may be less susceptible to falls.

Foods to avoid

As well as eating the right foods during menopause, you should avoid or reduce your intake of those that might make the symptoms worse. For instance, you should cut down on spicy foods, wine and caffeine, which many women find can provoke hot flushes or make them worse. Too much caffeine can also make you nervy and irritable and stop you sleeping properly, and may reduce your body's ability to use and store calcium. Cut down on

> **HELPFUL HERBS**
>
> A number of herbal remedies on the market are said to help relieve the symptoms of menopause, and may be worth trying, although there is no strong scientific basis for the effects claimed for them. They include red clover (*Trifolium pratense*), which is is rich in phyto-oestrogens; black cohosh (*Cimicifuga racemosa*) and blue cohosh (*Caulophyllum thalictroides*), which affect female sex hormone secretion; and liquorice (*Glycyrrhiza glabra*), chasteberry (*Vitex agnus-castus*), and the Chinese herb dong quai (*Angelica sinensis*). All are generally harmless when taken in moderation, but take care with liquorice—too much for too long can cause bowel problems, reduce levels of infection-fighting steroids, and cause high blood pressure.

your salt intake because a high salt intake will raise your blood pressure; and stop smoking—women who smoke tend to lose bone mass faster than nonsmokers.

Exercise and mood

Regular exercise, especially weight-bearing exercise such as walking, jogging and moderate weight training, will help to increase bone mass, improve your circulation, and help you to control your weight. It will also make you feel better because it triggers the release of endorphins, the pleasure-inducing hormones produced in your brain. The effects of these endorphins linger for several hours, improving your overall mood and helping to combat stress.

Weight-bearing exercise needs to be done about 3 to 4 times a week along with aerobic and flexibility activities.

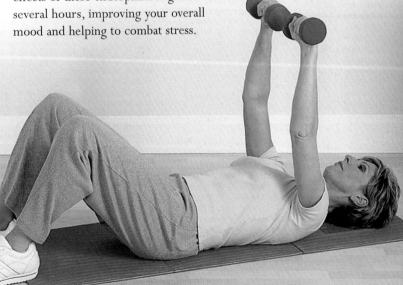

Viropause

There may or may not be such a thing as a male menopause (viropause), at least not in the way that menopause in women exists, but some men do seem to undergo some sort of change when they reach middle age. This is probably mostly psychological—regret for the loss of their youthful energy and ambitions, and for their declining physical and sexual abilities—but there also may be a hormonal basis.

Levels of testosterone, the male sex hormone, decline with age, and sexual problems such as a lessening of sexual interest (see page 76) and problems with erection and orgasm are commoner in

older men. This clear physical evidence of ageing and mortality can have a psychological effect, and combined with a sense of unfulfilled promise (or even of failure) it can induce a persistent low mood known as "involutional melancholia".

Low testosterone levels may also be associated with clinical depression that resists treatment until testosterone is given, either in the form of capsules or as skin patches, injections or implants. Such treatment works only if the testosterone is low in the first place, so a blood test is needed before it can be prescribed.

Prostate problems

As well as possibly suffering from low testosterone levels, middle-aged and elderly men can experience prostate problems. The prostate gland, found only in men, surrounds the outlet of the bladder and produces part of the seminal fluid. A common problem for older men is enlargement of the prostate, and cancer of the prostate is the commonest male cancer. Enlargement of the prostate gland can give rise to problems with urination, both in getting started ("urinary hesitancy") and in maintaining a good stream of urine (an early sign may be an inability to hit the porcelain of the urinal), and it can make it difficult to empty the bladder completely.

Medications such as dutasteride (Avodart) and finasteride (Proscar) can reduce the size of an enlarged prostate, but if left untreated even a benign (non-cancerous) enlargement of the prostate can cause painful retention of urine and may necessitate surgery. Unfortunately, the conventional medications and prostate surgery can both make any sexual problems worse. This is one reason why many men with prostate problems are

Sexual relationships between middle-aged men and women have been given a boost by the development of anti-impotence pills, which are some of the new millennium's wonder drugs.

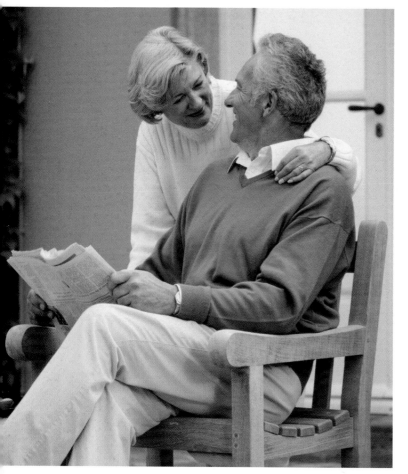

HERBS FOR PROSTATE PROBLEMS

Three herbal medicines appear to be effective for relieving prostate problems, especially mild to moderate prostatic enlargement, and they seem to be better tolerated than conventional medication. These herbs—saw palmetto (*Serenoa repens*), stinging nettle root (*Urtica dioica*), and pygeum bark (*Pygeum africanum*)—are better used in combination than alone.

Saw palmetto extract contains chemicals called sterols that probably counteract hormone-driven prostatic enlargement, and nettle root extract seems to work in a similar fashion. Pygeum has a more complex action, because as well as counteracting prostatic enlargement it seems to shrink the prostate and prevent the build-up of cholesterol.

The only significant potential problem with these medicines is that saw palmetto can cause inaccurate estimations of prostate-specific antigen (PSA) production. PSA is a protein produced in the prostate, and the level of PSA in the blood helps doctors to diagnose and monitor prostate problems. So if you are thinking of taking saw palmetto, it is wise to get your doctor to check your PSA before you start.

If you wish to look into herbal treatment further, seek the advice of a qualified herbalist (preferably a member of an appropriate professional body).

prey to unscrupulous purveyors of useless and expensive "snake oil" treatments purporting to help their sexual performance.

How diet can help

Through middle age and beyond, foods such as shellfish, meat and avocados may help enhance your sexual function, and vegetables and other foods containing plenty of protective antioxidant nutrients such as vitamins B, C and E can help to keep your prostate healthy.

Minerals such as zinc and selenium will help the antioxidants to function and will also boost your immune system, while lycopene (which gives tomatoes their red colour, and is found in other fruits and vegetables) concentrates in and protects your prostate.

Soya products such as tofu and soya milk, taken three or four times a week, and powdered soya protein sprinkled on cereals or mixed in cold drinks, can also protect your prostate as well as make an important contribution to your general health and wellbeing.

One of the oldest reputed aphrodisiacs, oysters can improve a man's sex life because they are high in zinc, which is essential for testosterone production.

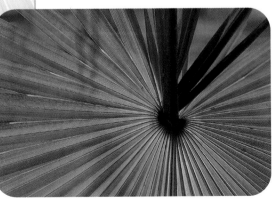

alcohol in the diet

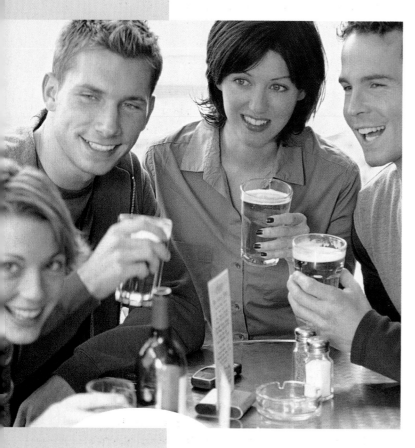

Alcoholic drinks are very much a mixed blessing. On the plus side, many people find that alcohol helps them to relax and to socialize, but on the negative side it can cause illness, accidents and antisocial behaviour including violence.

There is some evidence that alcohol taken in moderation may help to reduce the risk of heart attacks, but this only applies for men aged over 45 and women over 55. Younger people probably don't benefit from it, and anyway there are better ways to keep your heart in shape, such as eating a healthy diet, keeping your weight under control, not smoking, and taking plenty of exercise.

Food and drink

Alcohol has a number of potentially harmful effects on your body's ability to absorb and use many of the important nutrients in your food, especially vitamins and minerals. If you drink regularly, you should make sure that your diet is rich in these nutrients so that you do not become deficient in them.

Avoid processed foods, which tend to be low in important nutrients, and steer clear of saturated fats and fried foods because these can place an extra burden on your liver and gall-bladder, which are already overworked through coping with the alcohol. Cutting out these foods also will help you to reduce the intake of calories that you get from your food, to compensate for the extra calories you get from the alcohol.

To keep your vitamin intake high, eat plenty of fruit and leafy vegetables, whole grains, dried beans, nuts, lean meat and poultry. These will provide you with B-group vitamins such as B_1, B_5, B_6, B_{12},

did you know?

If you drink only in moderation and avoid "binge drinking", you should be able to enjoy the benefits of alcohol while avoiding its harmful effects. Official guidelines recommend that women have no more than one drink ("unit") a day and men no more than two—one drink is half a pint of beer, or a glass of wine, or a single shot of spirits. It is best to avoid alcohol in pregnancy.

and folate, and the antioxidant vitamins C and E that help to protect your liver from damage by the alcohol.

Drinkers, especially heavy drinkers, can easily become deficient in zinc, so your diet should include foods such as eggs, fish and shellfish, Brazil nuts, and almonds, which are rich in this mineral. The Brazil nuts and almonds also will boost your magnesium and iron levels, and you should keep your calcium levels high by eating cheese and other calcium-rich dairy products.

Finally, remember that alcohol is absorbed into your bloodstream far more quickly when your stomach is empty. It's a good idea to eat before you drink, or take drink only as an accompaniment to a meal, but beware of bar snacks such as salted nuts or potato crisps because they just make you more thirsty.

Social drinking

Controlling your intake of alcohol is not always easy when you are drinking in a social setting, whether it is an informal gathering of friends at home or at your local bar, a party, or a formal function. To avoid drinking too much, try to:

- decide in advance how much you want to drink, and stick to this limit;
- put your glass down between each sip, to help you drink more slowly;
- alternate between alcoholic and non-alcoholic drinks;
- don't be afraid to say "No" when you are offered a drink you don't want;
- remember that your willpower will be reduced by alcohol, so when you've had a few drinks you might lose your ability to resist having a few more.

DRINK PROBLEMS

Most people drink sensibly and in moderation, and their drinking tends to vary from time to time and place to place. For example, they may enjoy an occasional beer at lunch time or a cocktail after work, and a beer or a glass of wine with their evening meal.

The repertoire of dependent drinkers, however, is much narrower. Their drinking will be largely independent of their mood or the setting, and focused on the avoidance of withdrawal symptoms. Drinking becomes an addiction (see page 64) that dominates their lives, and the thought of the next drink becomes a preoccupation, just as an obsession with the next "hit" becomes dominant in a heroin or crack cocaine addict. Regular drinkers also usually develop a tolerance for alcohol, which allows them to drink more and still be able to function. This tolerance effect is at the centre of their physical dependence on alcohol, and sometimes as their tolerance for alcohol increases, so does their tolerance for other drugs such as tranquillizers.

The withdrawal symptoms may be very minor at first, but as time goes by they become steadily more severe, especially in the mornings, when the dependent drinker feels cravings for alcohol to make him or her feel better. These cravings are often the first warning sign the drinker notices, although he or she may deny their existence. At the same time, the person often becomes aware of his or her compulsion to drink, perhaps when he or she realizes that it is difficult to walk past an off-licence or a bar without going in and buying a drink.

Although some heavy drinkers are able to reduce their alcohol consumption to more "social" levels, for the majority of people with severe alcohol problems the only successful option is total abstinence.

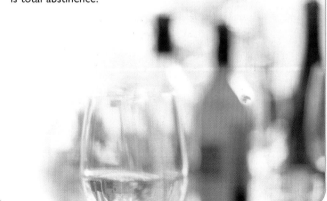

diet and smoking

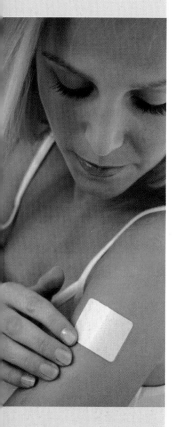

Any reasonably intelligent adult can list a whole series of reasons why smoking is bad, and cigarette packs in many countries carry dire and graphic warnings about the health consequences of smoking. These include emphysema and cancer, high blood pressure, heart and artery diseases, strokes, weakened bones, tooth and gum problems and impotence.

Yet many people continue to smoke. This is partly because, in some ways, tobacco is more addictive than heroin, and withdrawal from it is unpleasant (although seldom dangerous), and partly because there is also a degree of psychological dependence on it.

But the main obstacle to quitting is that people are unable to accept that the warnings apply to them; smokers tend to pay more attention to what they see as the "positive aspects". For instance, they may enjoy the taste of tobacco, or associate smoking with pleasant social situations, with "being sophisticated", or even with sex. They may find that it helps break the ice at social gatherings, or that it gives them something to do with their hands when they are not busy. Many people also smoke to reduce stress, and some people smoke because they think that it keeps their weight down.

All of these objections to quitting can be overcome if the will to do it is there, perhaps with the assistance of a nicotine replacement gum or patch. However, if you do not feel sufficiently motivated to quit, the first thing would be to motivate yourself properly. It is far better to try and quit when you feel sufficiently motivated, for then you will succeed.

Quitting smoking also can be helped by a number of techniques. Cognitive therapy involves understanding the pattern of your smoking, and you will be asked to keep a diary, listing every cigarette and the context in which you had it (what you were doing before lighting up, who you were with, etc.), so that you can identify the main triggers or cues of your habit. The aim then is to devise alternatives to the cigarette in response to that cue. If you are working with a therapist, each session involves an examination of your "homework" from the previous session, together with advice on how to improve.

Hypnotherapy is said to work by acting on the unconscious mind to

did you know?

Because smoking puts extra pressure on your cardiovascular system, avoid junk and processed foods, and reduce your salt intake because too much salt can promote high blood pressure. In addition, you should cut down on animal protein, apart from fish, and reduce your consumption of dairy products. This will help your heart and circulation by cutting the amount of saturated fat in your diet. It is also worth reducing your caffeine consumption if you are hoping to quit smoking. Too much caffeine will make you jittery and more likely to reach for a cigarette.

FATTER BUT FITTER

A common worry among smokers who want to give up is that they will rapidly put on weight. It's true that many ex-smokers gain weight, but their average increase is just 2.3 to 3.7 kg (5 to 8 pounds) and most lose that again within 2 to 5 years. And anyway, you would need to put on at least 34 kg (75 pounds) to cancel out the health benefits of quitting smoking.

To help yourself avoid weight gain when you become an ex-smoker, try following these simple tips:

- don't eat fatty or sugary high-calorie foods;
- if you feel like eating a snack between meals, do something else instead;
- if you must snack, eat fruit or raw vegetables;
- drink plenty of water instead of sweetened soft drinks;
- cut down your alcohol intake;
- take more exercise—it's much easier when you don't smoke.

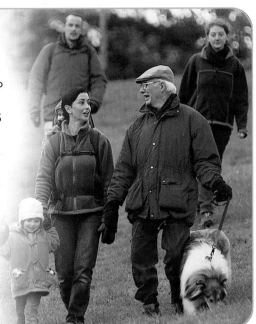

strengthen the willpower to quit or at least reduce the desire to smoke. Many people swear by it, although there is no objective evidence in scientific trials to prove that hypnotherapy is better than any other approach.

Where there's smoke...

Research carried out in the United States and many other countries around the world has shown that smokers tend to add to their health problems by eating poor diets. For example, they generally eat less fruit and vegetables than most nonsmokers. This leaves them deficient in the protective vitamins C, E, folate and betacarotene (the source of vitamin A) that could help reduce the damage to their body cells caused by the dangerous chemicals in tobacco smoke. It also means their intake of dietary fibre is less.

Another consequence of not eating enough fruit and vegetables is that smokers tend to fill up on fatty foods, and so they often have a higher intake of calories than nonsmokers. They are also likely to consume more alcohol than nonsmokers.

Compensatory eating

If you are a smoker, try and give it up. Meanwhile, make sure you are eating a healthy and balanced diet that includes plenty of the nutrients that can help counteract the harmful effects of smoking.

Make a determined effort to eat more fruit, especially oranges (or orange juice), berries, plums, and dark-green leafy vegetables plus beans, lentils, peas, green peppers, carrots and tomatoes. These are all good sources of vitamins and dietary fibre. You can boost your fibre and B-vitamin levels still further by eating whole-grain cereals, wholemeal bread, nuts (especially Brazil nuts) and brown rice. Onions and garlic are also helpful because they contain chemicals thought to help reduce the risk of cancer and heart disease.

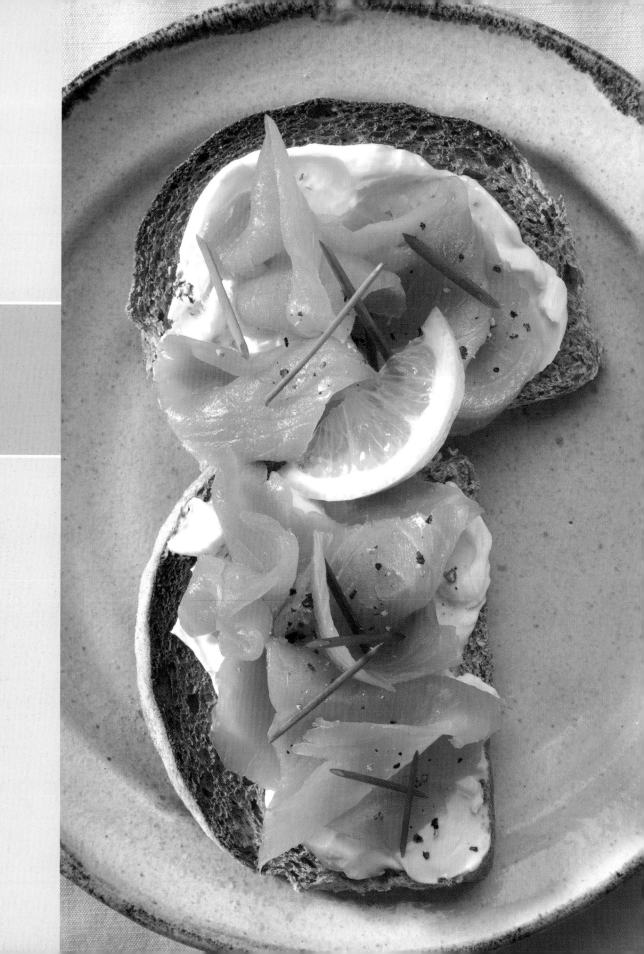

4

WHAT SHOULD I EAT FOR
A SPECIFIC PROBLEM?

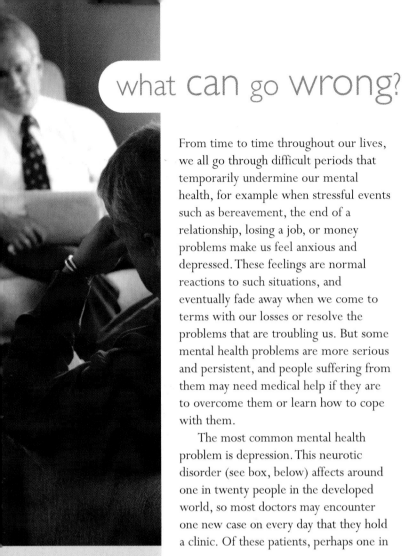

what can go wrong?

From time to time throughout our lives, we all go through difficult periods that temporarily undermine our mental health, for example when stressful events such as bereavement, the end of a relationship, losing a job, or money problems make us feel anxious and depressed. These feelings are normal reactions to such situations, and eventually fade away when we come to terms with our losses or resolve the problems that are troubling us. But some mental health problems are more serious and persistent, and people suffering from them may need medical help if they are to overcome them or learn how to cope with them.

The most common mental health problem is depression. This neurotic disorder (see box, below) affects around one in twenty people in the developed world, so most doctors may encounter one new case on every day that they hold a clinic. Of these patients, perhaps one in four hundred is referred to a psychiatrist, and one in one thousand needs to be admitted to hospital. These figures suggest that not only do the great majority of people with clinical depression not see a psychiatrist, but also that they receive little or no specific treatment of any kind.

Depression can occur at any time during life, including childhood, but it is perhaps commoner later in life. For instance, of all women who become depressed at some point in their lives, about half do so at around the time of their menopause, when they are in their late forties or early fifties.

More severe psychiatric disorders also can strike at any age, although the serious psychotic illnesses (see box, opposite) do not commonly occur after the age of about 35 or 40. Schizophrenia and bipolar affective disorder usually start during adolescence and early adulthood, but there are some conditions of old age that can resemble them. In later life,

neurotic disorders

Psychiatrists divide mental health problems into two main types, the neurotic disorders and the psychotic disorders. The neurotic disorders, by far the more common type, are basically more intense, long-lasting, and potentially harmful forms of negative thoughts and feelings that we all experience in a minor way from time to time. They include depression, anxiety states, phobias, compulsions, and obsessions.

In neurotic disorders, no matter how severe they are, there is always some grip on reality. For example, a person may be profoundly anxious, to the extent that he may feel entirely detached from his surroundings or even from his own body, but the individual doesn't feel with total conviction that he or his surroundings have literally changed.

what should I eat for a specific problem?

mental illnesses can arise from failing senses (for example, paranoid illness arising if a person persistently misinterprets his or her environment due to poor hearing or sight) but memory problems, including dementia, are the main psychiatric disorders.

Diagnosing a disorder

If you feel that your mental health is failing in some way, there are a few points you should consider before seeking medical help. The first is that psychiatric disorders or mental illnesses usually involve a pattern of symptoms rather than a single isolated symptom. For example, it is reasonably common for someone who is very tired or stressed to experience a simple hallucination, such as a loud noise or perhaps his or her name being called. And often someone who has suffered a bereavement may have brief hallucinations about the person who has died. These can include hearing the deceased person's key in the lock, or catching a brief glimpse of him or her in a crowded street. These isolated symptoms are part of normal experience during such stressful or fatiguing circumstances, and are not indicators of mental illness.

Similarly, if you are aware that you are forgetting things, then your forgetfulness is much more likely to be due to poor concentration, anxiety, or the natural effects of ageing than it is to any physical disorder of the brain. A diagnosis of dementia, for example, depends on a number of factors, of which memory problems are only one type.

It also is important to remember that the development of the symptoms of mental illness takes some time. It is, for instance, a very common experience to feel low in mood and wonder what is the point of doing anything. In general, this is

---

psychotic disorders

Usually much more severe than neurotic disorders, psychotic disorders are not rooted in normal thoughts and feelings. They include schizophrenia, psychotic depression, bipolar affective disorder (manic depression) and dementia. Psychotic illnesses are accompanied by a loss of contact with reality. For example, a person may develop fixed beliefs or delusions that she has special powers or that she has changed in some way. The person may develop hallucinations, which are her own thoughts, but she does not recognize them as such. For example, she might hear voices that she mistakenly believes come from outside, and belong to other people.

However, not everything a psychotic person does is motivated by, or is part of, her psychosis. For instance, the individual may be capable of deciding which brand of breakfast cereal to eat or even of making a legally valid will, despite having psychotic ideas about other areas of life.

---

a brief feeling lasting anything from a few minutes to a day or two. But if the low and pessimistic mood fails to lift (or gets worse) over a period of 10 to 14 days, this may indicate a developing clinical depression.

Knowing what can go wrong is important, but constantly being fearful that something *will* go wrong is unhealthy. The chances are that you will escape serious problems, and even if you don't, early treatment can often nip them in the bud. And there are things that you can do for yourself, such as following some of the dietary suggestions in this book, which have the potential to either prevent or minimize the impact of some of the problems.

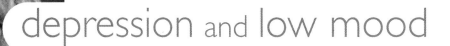

depression and low mood

Everybody has ups and downs. One of the problems in psychiatry is that we use several words in a clinical sense that also appear in everyday conversation. "Depression" is a classic example. People often say that they are "depressed" when they mean really that they are dissatisfied, unhappy, or fed up. Such feelings are a normal part of life; complex emotions are the price we pay for having complex and adaptive minds. The "bad" things balance the "good" things, and these feelings pass. To medicalize these normal vicissitudes of mood is wrong. We often behave as if we had an inalienable right to be happy all the time. We have not.

Clinical depression

If you are diagnosed as clinically depressed, it is quite different to just feeling unhappy. A pattern of low and deteriorating mood sets in over a week or so. It does not lift. Your outlook is pessimistic, and you feel (and look) sad, anxious, even panicky. You can feel cut off from others. You lose enjoyment in things, and may become irritable or overly sentimental.

Sometimes you may become pre-occupied with worries about death or even have suicidal thoughts. You may experience a profound lack of sexual interest and ability. Your sleep is

do you have a problem with depression?

Over at least the past week or two, have you

	YES	NO
Become tearful for no particular reason, or if someone says something nice to you, or if you see sentimental scenes on TV, for example?	☐	☐
Felt unduly anxious or panicky?	☐	☐
Regularly experienced broken sleep, either by persistent difficulty in getting off to sleep, or by frequent waking, or by waking un-refreshed (or all of these)?	☐	☐
Stopped enjoying things that usually give you pleasure?	☐	☐

	YES	NO
Had difficulty concentrating, even on a subject that would usually interest you?	☐	☐
Lost interest in sex?	☐	☐
Become more irritable?	☐	☐
Started to feel guilty, or a burden?	☐	☐
Started to cut yourself off from family and friends, or stopped socializing?	☐	☐
Felt hopeless about the future?	☐	☐

Answering "Yes" to more than one of these questions may mean that you are experiencing more than the normal transient periods of low mood, and that you should do something about it. If in any doubt, seek professional help.

what should I eat for a specific problem?

disturbed, often severely, and you have trouble both in getting off to sleep, and with waking throughout the night or during the early hours of the morning. Your whole thinking process can change, and put a negative spin on everything you do. A day when you get a promotion but burn the rice, would just be the day you burn the rice, thus proving yourself not just a bad cook, but a bad human being!

Clinical depression needs to be diagnosed professionally as it requires treatment of some kind. Mild forms may respond to "talking therapy", such as cognitive therapy, but in more severe cases, the burden of symptoms may be so pronounced that the individual only would benefit from medication.

Helping keep depression at bay

But, whether you are feeling "blue" or suffering from clinical depression, there is still much that you can do to help yourself. Diet is an important element to consider but there are other simple measures you can take to lift your spirits.

Low mood is often worse for being hidden. Talk to friends and family and try to spend less time alone; be as busy as possible. Exercise, preferably outdoors, as often as you can. Be aware of the present or try to take short views of life, a day, or a few hours, at a time. Try not to judge yourself. Learn to meditate, or study a relaxing discipline such as t'ai chi.

People often become more miserable as days shorten marking the approach of winter. For some, this becomes a pattern, and they are said to have SAD (seasonal affective disorder). Although not every-one accepts the existence of SAD as a psychiatric disorder, a seasonal onset of clinical depression is well established. The effect is mediated by the hormone melatonin. Melatonin (see page 14) is central to the control of the body's daily rhythms, including the sleep-wake cycle, and these rhythms are influenced by natural light.

Beta blockers, oral contraceptives, some antihypertensive drugs, steroids, and opiate painkillers, together with non-prescribed alcohol and recreational drugs, especially Ecstasy and cocaine, are often associated with depression. The commonest drug of all, caffeine, may not cause depression, but it can increase anxiety, and if you are feeling jittery, see how you feel after a week's abstinence from coffee or cola drinks.

DISPELLING SAD

Ordinary tungsten-filament light bulbs emit yellow light, without the other colours of the spectrum. Sunlight contains the full rainbow of colours to make white light. The intensity of the light is important, and can be duplicated by special, commercially available, light boxes. You sit in front of the box for 20–30 minutes per day. But light boxes are expensive and not everyone benefits from them.

To find out if you may benefit, you can buy a natural light bulb. They are more expensive than ordinary bulbs, and often last no longer, but installing one in the room that you most commonly use may help to lift your mood. Low-energy bulbs are no good here.

If the natural light bulb lifts the mood, then it may be worth investing in a light box.

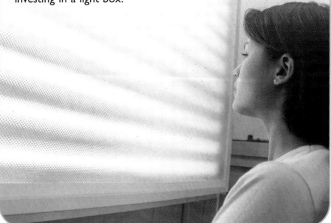

Selenium, zinc and chromium Although not in high doses, selenium (present in oysters, mushrooms, and above all, Brazil nuts), zinc (present in shellfish, seafood and eggs), and chromium (chromium picolinate) also have a demonstrable positive effect on low mood and on clinical depression.

S-adenosyl methionine (SAMe) in large doses (600 mg+ per day), is a very promising antidepressant. Studies have shown that it may be as good as commonly used antidepressants. It seems to have no major side effects, but it is expensive and has a short shelf life. SAMe 1,4-butanedisulphonate is the most stable form.

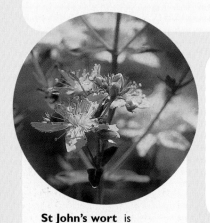

Very large doses of B vitamins (ten times the RDA), taken for a year, may improve general mental wellbeing, at least according to one widely quoted study from 1995. Apart from to your wallet, such large daily doses are thought to be reasonably safe, although irreversible sensory nerve damage may occur with too much vitamin B_6 (pyridoxine). Folic acid (folate) and vitamin B_{12} are vital to the breakdown of serotonin to form melatonin.

St John's wort is probably best for mild depression, or low spirits, rather than any more severe condition. While we do not know exactly how it works, one of its important constituents, hyperforin, has properties similar to the SSRI class of antidepressants (see page 12).

Eat folate-containing foods Folate does not in itself lift the mood but some people with clinical depression have low levels of it in the blood and there is good evidence that the effects of antidepressant drugs may be greatly reduced if folate levels are low. Folate-rich foods include fortified bread and cereals, strawberries, spinach, lettuce, citrus fruit and juice, avocado, peanuts, chickpeas, peas and broccoli. Folate levels in food decline with time, so the fresher, the better. Folate is lost in cooking water, so steaming or stir-frying is preferable.

Fish oils provide a hopeful avenue in the treatment of mood problems, including clinical depression. The specific form used to treat depression is omega 3 fatty acids in doses of 1 gram or more per day. How they work is a matter of debate; but we know that the compounds are involved in the structure and maintenance of cell membranes. Omega 3 fatty acids seem to help in bipolar affective disorder, especially in the depressive phase, and controlled trials of their use are underway.

mood changes after childbirth

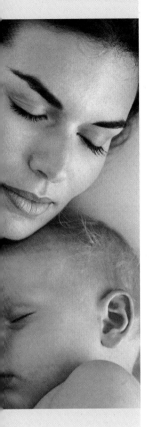

For most women, having a baby is a joyous event, but for many, the initial elation is followed by a gloomier spell called the baby blues. For some women, this gloom descends into postnatal depression, and a very small minority of new mothers suffer from a more serious condition, puerperal (or postnatal) psychosis. Although all of these psychiatric conditions have been ascribed to hormonal imbalances, it seems that only the baby blues are a direct consequence of the hormonal changes that occur after giving birth.

It is important to bear in mind that a woman is in particular need of sensitive support in the days and weeks after childbirth. The baby blues affect virtually all new mothers (up to 80 percent) within the first week after delivery, and last for only about two or three weeks. The condition is so common it probably should not be classed as a psychiatric disorder. It needs no specific medical treatment.

Postnatal depression affects between one in ten and one in five new mothers. It carries on beyond the first month after

symptoms of...

BABY BLUES

- mood swings
- sleep disturbance
- tiredness
- fatigue
- mild sadness
- tearfulness
- anxiety
- irritability
- increased sensitivity
- mild confusion

The great majority of women recover from these symptoms completely and are not at any greater risk of subsequently developing depression.

POSTNATAL DEPRESSION

- persistent low mood
- severe mood swings
- severe insomnia
- constant fatigue
- getting no pleasure from life
- emotional numbness
- feeling trapped
- withdrawing from family and friends
- lack of concern for yourself
- lack of concern for your baby
- excessive concern for your baby
- feelings of inadequacy or inability to cope

The symptoms of postnatal depression vary greatly from one woman to another. Postnatal depression is not something you can diagnose or treat yourself, so you should always seek medical advice.

self-help to beat the blues

Eat plenty of **fruit and vegetables** and protein-rich foods, particularly **fish**. Fish also contains essential fatty acids, minerals and iodine, and these, too, help stabilize your mood.

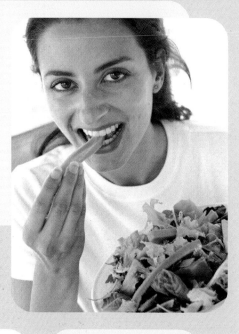

Cut down on **high-carbohydrate, sugary and processed foods** as these can increase levels of irritability and emotional fragility.

Reduce your **caffeine** intake and avoid **alcohol**. Drinking less caffeine will help to minimize mood swings, and alcohol is a depressant drug that will make them worse.

Eat frequent small meals, rather than three full meals a day. This is another way to ease mood swings because it will stabilize your blood sugar levels.

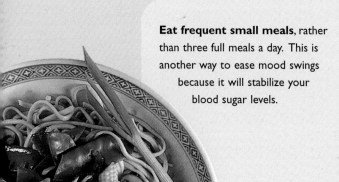

birth and the symptoms are indistinguishable from depression that can occur at other times (see page 54). As with other forms of depression, self-diagnosis is unwise and any woman who feels she may be suffering from it must seek medical advice.

Proper medical attention is also essential if puerperal psychosis is suspected, because it is a serious mental illness with severe symptoms constituting a loss of contact with reality. A woman with puerperal psychosis may experience severe depression, acute anxiety, chaotic or irrational thoughts or speech, paranoia, hysteria, hallucinations and may fear harming the baby or herself. Because of the detachment from reality, a woman suffering from it might not be aware that she is having problems so the responsibility for seeking medical help might fall on her family or friends. The condition, which affects perhaps one in a thousand new mothers, usually appears within six months of childbirth and is commonly part of a longer-standing psychotic illness.

How can diet help?

It is important to continue to eat well after giving birth, especially if you are breastfeeding (see pages 39–40).

A diet suitable for people with depression (see p. 56) will be helpful if you are suffering from postnatal depression, but you also can benefit from a modified diet if you have the baby blues. Make sure you include plenty of protein-rich foods in your diet as they are good sources of tryptophan, which can help to calm you and to improve your mood.

stress and burnout

Stress is not an illness and it is not a psychiatric diagnosis. Only post-traumatic stress disorder (PTSD) is an official psychiatric diagnosis, and even that is controversial. In Japan, however, karoshi (death from overwork stress) is becoming more widely recognized as a real, though difficult to prove, condition.

There is no blood test to measure the severity of a particular stress. We do know, however, its effects. Stress causes the release of hormones into the blood, which bring about the following actions: Breathing is speeded up, the rate and power of the heartbeat increases, the muscles benefit from increased blood flow, and blood is diverted from the gut, leading to the sensation of "butterflies in the stomach", or cramp if you have just eaten a large meal. Changes also occur to your blood sugar and hormone levels. The concept of stress as we think of it today dates from the work of Hans Selye. In 1956, he defined the stress response as having three distinct phases—"alarm" (where the body physically prepares for action), "resistance" (where the stress persists for longer, and some adaptation occurs) and "collapse" (where an intolerable, prolonged or often-repeated stress results in exhaustion).

None of us can avoid stress and its effects are very individual. Something that causes you considerable anxiety and upset may be taken in stride by another. There is scientific evidence to show that some stress improves performance; but after a point—which varies from person to person—increasing stress simply reduces it. So some stress is beneficial.

If you think you are suffering from stress, for example if you've taken the test on page 60 and scored 11 or more, contact your doctor or occupational health department. Although these symptoms suggest probable stress, they also may represent a physical illness, especially if they arise suddenly.

Managing stress

Stress may lower your body's resistance and make you more vulnerable to infection and illness, but there are things you can do to add beneficial nutrients to your diet to help boost your immune system. These are set out on page 61. You also should avoid alcohol and cigarettes. Alcohol interacts with many supplements and depletes nutrients. Nicotine increases the symptoms of anxiety and stress. Also, smoking induces an increased need for vitamin C and lower intakes of vitamin B_{12} and folic acid.

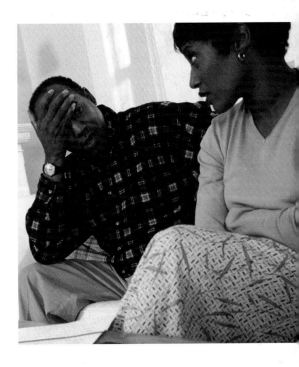

What if I am taking medication?

There are no prescribed drugs that specifically cater for stress. However, many people with stress may receive antidepressants or drugs designed to help anxiety (anxiolytics), such as propranolol or benzodiazepines (diazepam and drugs like it; buspirone). Some may be prescribed sleeping tablets (hypnotics).

The main concern is that most of these drugs may affect weight, glucose handling or both. This is not usually major, but it pays to watch your weight. If you are taking older-style antidepressants (clomipramine), diazepam, or buspirone you also should probably avoid grapefruit juice, especially. There are clinically significant interactions.

could you be suffering from stress and burnout?

	YES	NO
1 I sleep for 6 hours or more at least 4 nights a week.	☐	☐
2 My weight is about right for my height.	☐	☐
3 My smoking has increased lately.	☐	☐
4 I need an alcoholic drink when I return from work and/or to help me sleep.	☐	☐
5 I feel anxious every day before going to work, but OK at weekends and holidays.	☐	☐
6 I have no influence or control over my workload or the way I do my work.	☐	☐
7 I feel emotionally drained most of the time.	☐	☐
8 I get little or no recognition for my efforts.	☐	☐
9 I have at least one close friend with whom I can discuss personal matters.	☐	☐

	YES	NO
10 I have to neglect my family and friends because of work.	☐	☐
11 I spend 2 hours or more per day travelling to and from work.	☐	☐
12 I have enough income to meet my basic needs.	☐	☐
13 I regularly do something just for fun.	☐	☐
14 I regularly give and receive affection.	☐	☐
15 I give more than I ever get in return.	☐	☐
16 It seems as if I never see my house in daylight!	☐	☐
17 I do not have enough time to do my job.	☐	☐
18 If I am angry about something, I just let it out.	☐	☐
19 My job offers me little intellectual satisfaction.	☐	☐

Score 1 for 'Yes', and 0 for 'No' (except for questions 1, 2, 9, 12, 13, 14, 15, 19, where 'Yes' scores 0, and 'No' scores 1). A score of 11 or more means that you may be very highly stressed; 7–10 means that you need to look out that things do not worsen; 4–6 means that things are reasonably OK, but you should not be complacent; 0-3 shows that you have got the balance right—for now!

what should I eat for a specific problem?

self-help to calm down

Supplements and herbal teas People under long-term stress seem to be more prone to infection, and it may be worth taking zinc and vitamin C supplements to help boost the body's immunity. Camomile and mint teas will exert a calming effect on many people.

Cut down on caffeine One of the commonest drugs in regular use, caffeine, is taken in coffee, tea and cola drinks. It is addictive, though not as much as nicotine. Too much caffeine increases the symptoms of anxiety and can interfere with sleep. You may be surprised at how much better you feel if you significantly cut down, or cut out altogether, your caffeine consumption for about two weeks. If you already drink lots of coffee or cola, you may suffer withdrawal symptoms, such as headaches or craving for a week or so after quitting caffeine. But the symptoms soon pass.

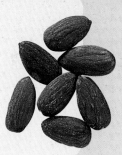

Foods with a low glycaemic index which release their sugars very slowly are the most helpful in combating stress. Choose whole-grain bread, vegetables, beans, buckwheat and oatmeal. These foods help to maintain a constant sugar level in the blood, thus ensuring that mood also stays constant. Foods with a high glycaemic index (see page 29) contain a lot of sugar that is released quickly. While they are very effective as short-term mood boosters, they have a transient effect and a rebound dip in mood is common. Fluctuations in sugar levels can have an adverse effect on mood, as well as playing havoc with a balanced diet (see stress and obesity, page 62).

Nuts, fruit and fish Almost all nuts but especially almonds and Brazil nuts, fruit and fish are rich in the B vitamins, especially B_3, B_5 and B_6; selenium; omega 3 fatty acids and taurine. All can be very beneficial in helping the symptoms of stress.

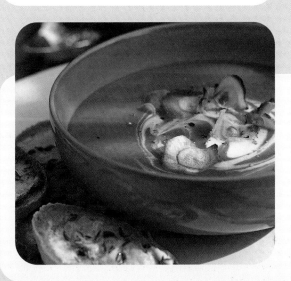

Eat comforting foods rather than indulging in comfort eating. A home-made soup on a cold day, for instance, may remind you of being cared for in childhood. A steaming bowl of porridge, scented with cinnamon and sweetened with raisins, can sustain you through the toughest day.

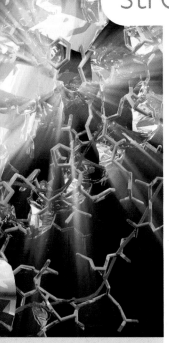

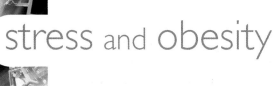

stress and obesity

Few people can be unaware that obesity is one of the greatest public health challenges facing us today. Its effects on physical health are known to include diabetes, heart disease, high blood pressure, stroke, gall-bladder problems, joint disease and even some cancers.

To be obese means to be too heavy for one's frame. Obesity is defined as a BMI (body mass index) of 30 or more, roughly a waist size of greater than 40 inches (102 cm) in men or 35 inches (89 cm) in women. Body mass is your weight in pounds divided by the square of your height in inches multiplied by 703.

Causes of obesity

The main cause of obesity is taking in more energy (calories) than you expend. Despite the assertions of different dietary schools of thought, it appears that diets high in fat and carbohydrates (including sugars), where there is no balance between fat and fibre intake, are more likely to result in obesity than diets where protein, fat, carbohydrate and fibre are in balance.

It is also the case that some people use energy from food faster than others. Most of us know someone who appears to be able to eat all the cakes and burgers he or she wishes without putting on weight, whereas you may only need to "look at" food to put weight on. The latter situation, however, may have some evolutionary value; the individual who is able to make the most of available food by turning it into fat may be the one who passes on his or her genes by surviving lean periods of food supply.

Genetic inheritance appears to be an important cause of obesity; some say as much as 80 percent. Certainly, if you have an obese identical twin, you are much more likely to be so too, than if you had a non-identical twin, brother, sister or parent who was obese.

Finally, psychological and personality factors can play an important role in obesity. Binge eating disorder, for instance, is much more common in obese people, and contributes both to the cause and outcome of the condition. While depression (see page 54) is classically associated with weight loss, weight gain is also common, especially in children who become depressed. More than half of people who are referred for surgery for severe obesity are clinically depressed; a threefold increase compared with the general population. The body's response to chronic stress may be part of the picture, but nobody yet knows for sure.

Leptin, a hormone involved with appetite suppression, is thought by some scientists to have the potential to create a miracle drug for obesity.

did you know?

Stress is frequently the culprit behind poor eating habits. In an effort to save time or energy, many people just grab whatever is available, such as sweets, potato crisps, cakes and biscuits. Typically, these are high in sugar or salt, and when eaten in excess lead to obesity. Unfortunately, stress also can make sticking to a slimming diet difficult, so most reputable weight-loss programmes also include an element of behaviour modification.

what should I eat for a specific problem?

The stress connection

During times of stress, certain hormones, especially glucocorticoids, are released into the blood. Glucocorticoids are involved in Cushing's disease (too much glucocorticoids) and Addison's disease (too little) and in each case have an effect on weight. As these hormones mediate our body's response to stress, the possibility exists that stress also may play a part in obesity. It seems that, in rats at any rate, the body's response to prolonged stress is reduced by taking energy-rich foods. Stressed rats calm down if they eat sugar. In other words, energy-rich food can be a stress-buster. Although the research was performed on rats, the results are consistent with what we already know about human behaviour. It fits in well with the common observation that a sweet, pleasurable food can temporarily calm a person down.

But the problem with using energy-rich food as a stress-buster, is that you have to know when to stop eating. You increase your abdominal energy stores, but you also get fat.

Knowing when to stop eating is regulated in the hypothalamus, deep in the brain, and in a "satiety centre" in the brain stem, just above the level of the spinal cord. The hormone leptin is an important player in this complex system. Leptin is produced in fatty tissue and effectively switches off appetite and increases energy consumption.

In normal weight, there is a balance between energy intake and expenditure. If the food supply is reduced, and body fat decreases, leptin levels will fall, so that there is both an increased need for food, and a reduced rate of metabolism. The sexual hormones close down, too. If there is an increase in body fat, leptin increases, appetite is reduced, and energy burned off more rapidly. Obesity occurs when the leptin system no longer exerts this fine control. Leptin deficiency is a rare (1–2 percent) cause of severe obesity.

Obesity as such is not usually associated with specific psychiatric symptoms, at least in adults. However, many obese people suffer from low self-esteem and social discrimination.

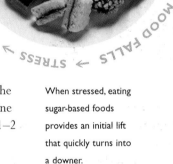

MOOD RISES → BLOOD SUGAR LEVEL FALLS ↘ MOOD FALLS ← STRESS ← EAT SUGARY FOOD ↑

When stressed, eating sugar-based foods provides an initial lift that quickly turns into a downer.

beneficial substitutions

REPLACE	WITH
Sweets, biscuits and cakes	Fresh fruit or pieces of raw vegetables
Coffee, tea, cola drinks	Decaffeinated beverages, fruit juice or water
Beef, lamb and pork	Poultry and fish
Cheddar and other hard cheeses	Cottage, low-fat and goat's cheese
Fatty and fried food	Meat that has its visible fat cut away and is cooked with mono- or polyunsaturated oils

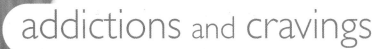

addictions and cravings

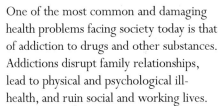

One of the most common and damaging health problems facing society today is that of addiction to drugs and other substances. Addictions disrupt family relationships, lead to physical and psychological ill-health, and ruin social and working lives.

Addictions as such are not mental illnesses. Strictly speaking, having an addiction means that your body has become physically dependent upon a substance, such as alcohol, nicotine, tranquillizers, barbiturates, opiates and other illicit drugs, or on the fumes from chemicals such as solvents or glues.

However, the concept of psychological addiction is often used to explain some forms of addiction-like behaviours, which are in fact poorly resisted compulsions or habits, rather than addictions in the true sense.

Compulsive gambling, stealing, shopping, or even, controversially, sex, fall into this category. The "addict" may find the compulsion irresistible, but although there is no question of physical dependence, recent research suggests that chemical systems within the brain, especially those using the neuro-transmitter dopamine (see page 16), may be heavily involved in maintaining these compulsions and cravings.

Kicking the habit

Getting free of an addiction is difficult and painful for most people. Medical advice and assistance is often desirable, and is essential for serious problems such as heroin addiction. But you cannot change unless the pain of staying as you are is greater than the pain of changing,

could you be having a problem with alcohol?

An alcoholic drink or two can help you to relax, and makes you feel good by boosting levels of the neurotransmitter dopamine in your brain. But excessive alcohol disrupts the normal functioning of your brain and nervous system. Habitual heavy drinking can also cause long-term mental and physical damage, disrupt your relationship with family and friends, and cause problems at work.

	YES	NO
1 Have you ever felt you should cut down on your drinking?	☐	☐
2 Have people annoyed you by criticizing your drinking?	☐	☐
3 Have you ever felt bad or guilty about your drinking?	☐	☐
4 Have you ever had a drink first thing in the morning (an "eye-opener") to steady your nerves or to get rid of a hangover?	☐	☐

This test assesses your dependence on alcohol, and it's called the CAGE questionnaire. It gets this name from the initial letters of key phrases and words in the questions —"cut down" (in question 1), "annoyed" (2), "guilty" (3), and "eye-opener" (4). Ninety percent of people with alcohol problems answer "yes" to one of these.

what should I eat for a specific problem?

and finding the pain of change unbearable is the commonest reason why people cannot shake their addictions.

How can diet help?

Firstly, a healthy, balanced diet will help you cope better with the initial high-stress period of quitting and will also improve your general physical and mental health—poor nutrition is common in people with addictions, and addicts are usually malnourished. An alcoholic, for example, gets most of his or her energy from alcohol, not from a balanced diet.

The second way that diet can help is by making it easier for you to cope with the withdrawal symptoms and cravings. Stress-busting foods (see page 61), especially those rich in vitamin B, calcium and magnesium, are important aids to overcoming the physical stresses of addiction, and calcium and magnesium may reduce the tremors that often accompany withdrawal. Fatty acids, found in foods such as oily fish and in supplements such as the oil of the evening primrose (*Oenothera biennis*), are not only helpful for maintaining general nutrition but also may reduce withdrawal symptoms, while foods containing zinc, vitamin C and other antioxidants help to protect the liver and boost resistance to infection.

Foods rich in tryptophan (see page 13), and the supplement 5-hydroxy tryptophan (5HTP), may also reduce stress and mitigate the symptoms of withdrawal. Their antidepressant actions can be especially helpful in the rebound depression that is so common in cocaine withdrawal. Eating foods rich in inositol (see page 28) is also recommended.

self-help to beat the blues

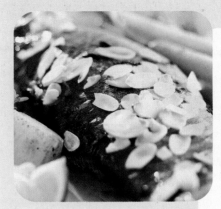

Eat plenty of stress-busting foods, particularly nuts, fruit and fish, which are rich in the B vitamins (Brazil nuts and almonds also have useful amounts of beneficial magnesium), and cheese and other calcium-rich dairy products.

Supplements: Fish oils and the oil of the evening primrose are both helpful for reducing withdrawal symptoms, while zinc and vitamin C can help boost the body's immunity and protect the liver.

Herbs: Siberian ginseng and valerian are said to be helpful with combating withdrawal symptoms.

can we become addicted to foods?

People can develop strong cravings for certain foods, although that doesn't necessarily mean that they become physically addicted to them. Some studies suggest that an excess of sugary or fatty foods can switch off our natural appetite suppressor, the hormone leptin, with the result that we eat much more of these foods than is good for us.

In addition, the brain uses glucose as its energy supply and a "hit" of sugar can lift the mood for a brief period. Sugar also can increase the uptake of tryptophan into the body, again with a mood-elevating effect, and fats have a similar though less powerful action. Most of us prefer pleasure to pain, so it is easy to see how this is an experience that we may wish to repeat. And because many foods, especially fast foods, are loaded with sugars and fats to give them extra taste, cravings for the pleasurable sensations produced by them are common.

eating disorders

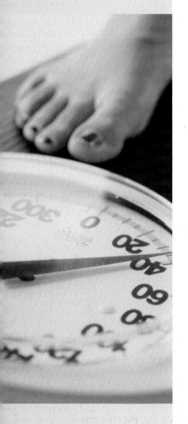

Eating disorders are extremely common throughout the world. There is a growing epidemic of obesity, and in developed countries binge eating, bulimia nervosa, and anorexia nervosa are also major health problems. These eating disorders are more common in females than in males but they generally have a worse outcome in males, perhaps because they are less well recognized or understood.

Eating disorders appear to result from a combination of psychological, relationship and social problems that lead to a preoccupation with food and weight. Although anorexia and bulimia are commonly associated with the young, older people may show similar obsessions with their weight. Some may become compulsive dieters, while others become obsessed with cosmetic surgery. When someone believes that his or her value as a person depends on how she or he looks, there will always be a risk of developing an eating disorder.

Binge eating and bulimia
Binge eating is a repeated, irresistible compulsion to eat very large amounts of food in relatively short periods of time,

usually an hour or two. This is almost always coupled with a feeling of being out of control of the eating, and the food may often be something as simple as an entire loaf of bread—the aim is the quantity of consumption rather than the nature of what is eaten. It is probably the most common eating disorder, and its sufferers may be overweight, normal weight, or even underweight.

Bulimia includes binge eating, but by no means everyone who experiences binge eating has bulimia. People who have bulimia do other things as well as binge-eat, such as making themselves vomit or using laxatives and diuretics to purge away the excess food, or taking excessive exercise to keep their weight down. The abnormal behaviour occurs frequently, often more than once a day, but is not always equally severe.

Anorexia nervosa
Very uncommon outside Western cultures, anorexia nervosa has been described by some authorities as a "culture-bound" disorder. Adolescent females in the West are bombarded with images of the "ideal" body shape and size, and although there have been some changes in the world of fashion it is still more usual to see models who are light and thin rather than broad and heavy.

Anorexia is essentially a phobia of gaining weight. People with anorexia are unable to maintain their weight and, typically, lose more than 15 percent of their normal body weight. Their image of their own bodies is distorted, and they will feel quite sincerely that they are fat even if objectively they are very thin. They often will vehemently deny that

symptoms of...
BINGE EATING

- eating what is clearly an unusually large amount of food, even when you are not really hungry
- eating much more quickly than usual during binge episodes
- eating until you are uncomfortably or even painfully full
- eating alone to conceal the problem from other people
- feeling that your eating is out of control
- feeling disgusted or guilty after overeating.

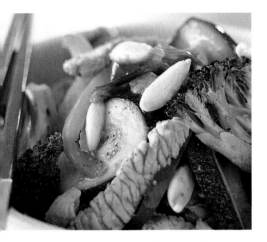

there is a problem, and work out many ways of persuading people that this is the case. Anorexics also may be very aware, almost to the last calorie, of the energy content of their food. Paradoxically, they may be keen cooks and do all the family cooking, making sure, of course, that they do not eat the food themselves.

How can diet help?
The treatment of bulimia can be difficult, and usually requires specialist help including psychotherapy, treatment with antidepressants, and guidance from a dietitian. Vitamin supplements help correct the nutritional imbalance that often results, and foods rich in zinc and calcium have a calming effect and increase appetite. Protein-rich foods can be helpful, because relatively small portions are enough to create a feeling of fullness or satisfaction and they are good sources of mood-enhancing trytophan. Junk foods and sugar should be avoided completely, and caution should be taken about eating carbohydrates in general.

Persuading anorexics to gain weight is not easy, and may require specialist assistance with psychotherapy as an important component. However, some research suggests that zinc supplements

may not only boost mood in anorexia, but also enhance weight gain. There are arguments both for and against this theory, and it does not mean that zinc deficiency causes anorexia.

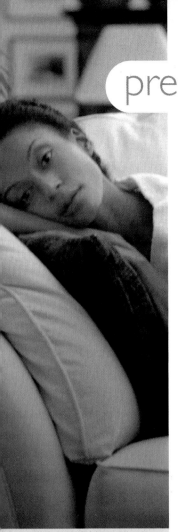

premenstrual syndrome

If you are a woman who dreads the onset of her monthly periods, you are not alone. As many as four out of every five women feel some unpleasant psychological or physical symptoms before each menstrual period, and about half of those experience symptoms severe enough to amount to the condition called premenstrual syndrome (PMS). And a small number of women, about one in twenty, suffer from premenstrual dysphoric disorder (PMDD), in which the symptoms are so severe that they badly disrupt the women's working and social lives (see box right).

The idea of the existence of PMS and PMDD has been controversial, with many arguing that it's wrong to make a disease out of a normal experience, and that the concept of PMS and PMDD says as much about the position of women in society as it does about the presence of an illness. Those who oppose the concept point out that there are no objective signs such as blood tests that are diagnostic of PMS and PMDD, and there is no evidence of any disruptive hormonal imbalance in the body. However, it does appear that the hormonal system connecting the brain with the pituitary gland and the ovaries (the hypothalamic-pituitary-gonadal, or HPG, axis) is closely involved.

Activity in the HPG axis seems to cause changes in the brain that lead to the symptoms of PMS and PMDD. The HPG axis is closely linked to the serotonin system and drugs that increase serotonin levels have been used successfully to treat both conditions. But many women rightly prefer to try a more natural approach first, and such an approach can include nutrients and supplements.

How can diet help?

In general, around the time of menstruation you should eat plenty of whole-grain bread and cereals to help keep your blood glucose levels stable, and foods rich in serotonin-boosting tryptophan, such as turkey, that may help relieve the symptoms of PMS and PMDD by capitalizing on the linkage between the hormonal system and serotonin. There is also good evidence that calcium and magnesium may be effective treatments if you take them in high enough doses.

symptoms of...
PMS & PMDD

PMS
- mild psychological discomfort
- breast tenderness
- bloating (with or without weight gain)
- swelling of hands and feet
- feeling emotionally brittle and easily upset
- sleep disturbance
- tiredness
- forgetfulness
- clumsiness
- increased irritability
- feelings of poor self-image

PMDD
- severe symptoms of PMS
- very low mood
- anxiety or tension
- severe mood swings
- significantly increased irritability

Although it is possible to get large quantities from your diet, especially from dairy products and seaweed (high in calcium) and green vegetables, nuts and seeds (rich in magnesium), many women find it easier to take supplements. Be careful, though, because too much calcium increases the risk of kidney stones. You can reduce this risk, although not eliminate it, by taking your calcium supplement immediately after a meal to slow down its absorption into your system.

It's also worth noting that a diet high in protein or refined foods can increase the amounts of calcium and magnesium that leave your body in your urine. If you suffer from PMS or PMDD, it might be wise to cut down on protein and refined foods while the symptoms last.

Vitamin B$_6$, which helps the formation of serotonin from tryptophan, is another nutrient that may be effective in combating PMS and PMDD, especially when taken with magnesium.

A popular herbal remedy is the oil of the evening primrose (*Oenothera biennis*), which is rich in omega 6 fatty acids (see page 24). Most women get adequate amounts in their normal diets and while there is not much scientific evidence that taking more has any measurable effect, it seems reasonably harmless and it has gained a good reputation for easing breast tenderness.

Another herb, chasteberry (*Vitex agnus-castus*), is widely used in Europe for treating the symptoms of PMS, PMDD and menopause. It appears to work by stimulating the production of dopamine (see page 16) in the brain, and by suppressing the sex hormone FSH (follicle stimulating hormone). The research evidence is not all that convincing but, like evening primrose oil, chasteberry may be worth trying.

self-help for less painful periods

Supplements: Increase your calcium and magnesium intake to around 1200 mg calcium and 350 mg magnesium.

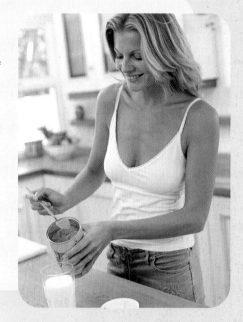

Eat plenty of foods rich in tryptophan such as turkey, chicken, fish, beans and soya products.

Increase your intake of vitamin B$_6$ by eating wheatgerm, oily fish (such as salmon and mackerel) and nuts.

To stabilize your mood, you should **avoid or cut down on caffeine and alcohol**, which can aggravate anxiety and irritability, and on sweet, sugary foods such as chocolate, which can affect your mood by making your blood sugar levels fluctuate.

You could try a herbal remedy, such as evening primrose or chasteberry. Both are claimed to relieve PMS symptoms such as breast tenderness.

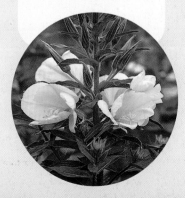

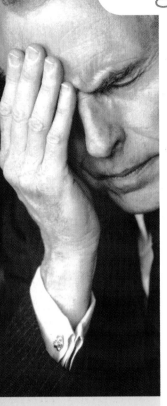

migraine

Migraines are more than just severe headaches. The throbbing, sickening pain they cause, usually on one side of the head or face, can be accompanied by a temporary loss of voice, general weakness or numbness, nausea, a painful sensitivity to light, and visual disturbances such as flashing lights or zigzag patterns. Migraines commonly start during the teenage years and may run in families. They affect up to 10 percent of the population and are 3.5 times more common in women than in men—an estimated 16 percent of menstruating women suffer from them.

Migraines do not always follow the same pattern, but they often build up slowly and last for a few hours or even a day or more. The throbbing quality is thought to be due to widening and increased pulsation of the arteries

supplying the scalp and face (the external carotid arteries) or the brain (the internal carotid arteries).

Migraines may be triggered by many different situations or events. Triggers tend to be individual to the person concerned, but the most common include stress, menstruation, sleep disturbance, a missed meal, or certain foods (see box, below). Sometimes, environ-mental factors such as bright or flickering lights or loud noise can act as triggers.

Preventing a migraine by avoiding known triggers, or treating it with painkillers or antimigraine drugs while it is still in its early stages, is generally more effective than treating the developed episode. Then, often the only the only thing that helps is to rest in a darkened room and wait for the headache to pass.

Can diet help?

Apart from identifying and avoiding trigger foods, the scientific evidence that diet can help is not strong. In principle, though, foods containing nutrients that boost the circulation should be effective—at least staving off an attack—provided such foods are not among those that can trigger your migraines.

For example, calcium and magnesium help reduce widening of the carotid arteries by improving the tone of the tiny

did you know?

The foods that can set off a migraine attack vary from one person to another, but these are among the most common and should be avoided.

- dairy products
- chocolate
- eggs
- citrus fruits
- meat and fish
- wheat and wheat products
- nuts and peanuts
- tomatoes
- onions
- corn and corn products
- apples
- bananas
- red wine
- monosodium glutamate
- pickled or cured foods
- artificial sweeteners

Keep a diary if you suffer from migraines but you aren't sure what is triggering them. Note down everything you eat or drink each day (including dressings and garnishes). If you suspect that environmental factors, such as noise or air pollution, might be responsible, make a note of your exposure to these as well. The diary will help you to link your migraine attacks to foods or events that preceded them, and identify possible triggers.

The herb feverfew (*Chysanthemum parthenium*) has been used for hundreds of years as a remedy for fever and headache and can help relieve migraine. It should not be taken by pregnant women, and will not work for everyone, but it is worth trying.

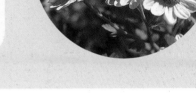

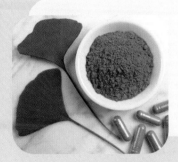

Circulation-boosting supplements and herbs may help to prevent an attack. Calcium, magnesium, lecithin, and ginkgo biloba all do this. Tryptophan-rich foods also may help to prevent and reduce attacks.

muscles in their walls, so supplements or foods rich in these substances can help. And for some people, foods rich in tryptophan may help to prevent and relieve attacks. This is because tryptophan reproduces something of the action of triptans, which increase brain serotonin and are the most effective orthodox antimigraine drugs currently available.

Ginkgo extract, made from the leaves of the ginkgo tree (*Ginkgo biloba*), is another substance that can improve the circulation and help to prevent attacks, and some sufferers may be helped by taking circulation-boosting lecithin granules.

When in doubt…

Consult your doctor about possible interactions between any supplements you take and prescribed medication.

when should you see a doctor?

If you have never suffered from migraine and you start getting severe, persistent, or recurrent headaches, you should consult your doctor without delay. And if you suffer any of the following types of headache you should seek prompt medical attention because they may be symptoms of potentially serious problems:

• sudden severe headache
• sudden severe headache and a stiff neck
• sudden severe headache and sensitivity to light
• headache after a blow to the head
• headache and confusion or blackouts
• headache and convulsions
• headache and fever
• headache and ear or eye pain

sleep problems

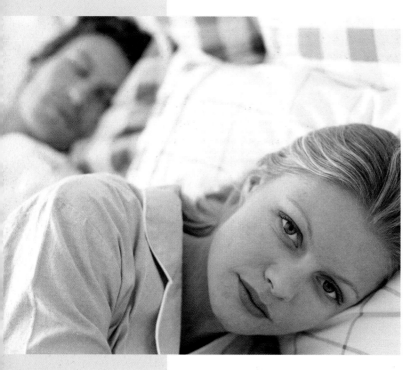

did you know?

We tend to sleep less during the summer months than we do during the winter, and less during hot weather than in cold. This is mainly because the extension of the normal day length by artificial means, such as candles and electric light, is comparatively new in our evolutionary history. As a species, we are much more used to a rhythm where the day begins at dawn and ends more or less at dusk, and our cycle of sleeping and waking is controlled by the action of the hormone melatonin (see page 14).

Few common disorders have as much impact on your quality of life than sleep problems. Being unable to sleep properly is frustrating in itself, and not getting enough sleep can make you irritable and drowsy during the day, impair your memory, and hamper your ability to concentrate on your work or to enjoy your leisure. And it can have more serious consequences if drowsiness makes you fall asleep at the wheel.

The amount of sleep that people need each night varies from person to person, but if you wake reasonably refreshed in the morning and are able to complete your day without undue sleepiness, then you are probably getting enough. The average for an adult is about eight hours, but this declines with age and many elderly people need only a few hours.

Causes of sleeplessness

Eating a heavy meal shortly before bedtime can make sleeping difficult, but going to bed on an empty stomach can be just as bad (see self help box, opposite).

We often sleep less if we are anxious or excited about something, but sleeplessness of this kind is usually temporary and it stops when the underlying reason is removed or resolved.

Restless leg syndrome (RLS) is an annoying disorder in which you are repeatedly woken by unpleasant tingling or painful sensations in your legs, which make you want to jerk or twitch your legs to relieve the discomfort.

If you continually suffer from poor sleep, however, it may be because your bed is too hard or too soft and there may be too much light or heat in your bedroom. You need to make sure your bed is comfortable and your bedroom is not too hot, too cold, or too light. You also should adopt a regular routine—try to go to bed and get up at the same times every day. Finally, don't read or watch television too much in bed.

How can diet help?

If you want a late-night snack you should avoid foods such as cured meats, mature cheeses, chocolate, pickles, and tomatoes, and red wine. These contain tyrosine, from which your brain makes the stimulating neurotransmitters dopamine and norepinephrine.

If you suffer from RLS, extra magnesium may also help as can the B-group vitamins (from, for example, whole grains), vitamin E (from wheatgerm), and iron (good sources include nuts, seeds and beans). Reducing your evening caffeine intake might also reduce the severity of RLS, but you should cut down on caffeine anyway because its stimulating effects will tend to keep you awake.

Sleeping pills

Although sleeping pills can sometimes be helpful, it's much better to avoid taking them if at all possible. They are drugs of dependence, which means that you need to increase the dose to maintain the same effect as time goes by, and you may suffer withdrawal symptoms when you stop taking them. And there is increasing evidence that taking sleeping pills regularly can reduce your general reaction times and increase your likelihood of being involved in an accident.

Mild antihistamine drugs sold as alternatives to sleeping pills can help you sleep, but if you take them for too long they can have unwanted side effects and may interact with prescription drugs.

A number of herbal remedies, taken as infusions, may help to promote sound sleep. Those containing extracts of plants such as hops (*Humulus lupulus*), passionflower (*Passiflora incarnata*), and valerian (*Valeriana officinalis*) are recommended.

Avoid caffeine, alcohol and nicotine for at least four hours before you go to bed and don't drink too much liquid during the late evening because it will fill your bladder and disturb your sleep.

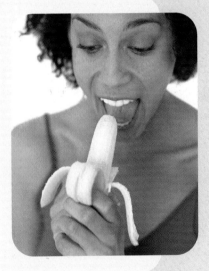

Eat a light snack shortly before bedtime, and the traditional glass of warm milk and a few biscuits works well because the milk contains sleep-inducing tryptophan (see page 13). As an alternative (especially if you don't like warm milk), try a snack based on other foods rich in tryptophan such as bananas, turkey, tuna or peanut butter.

To prevent leg cramps, increase your daily intake of calcium (found in dairy products), zinc (found in Brazil nuts and seafood), and magnesium (from nuts).

Try to exercise for 20 to 30 minutes during the day (for instance by brisk walking).

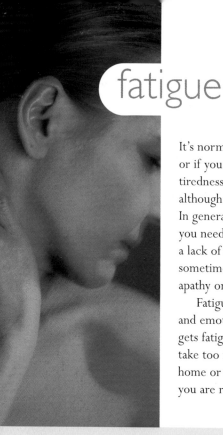

fatigue

It's normal to feel tired after a busy day, or if you haven't slept properly, but tiredness is not the same as fatigue, although it is often one of its symptoms. In general, tiredness is simply a sign that you need sleep, while fatigue is essentially a lack of energy and motivation sometimes combined with feelings of apathy or indifference.

Fatigue is a common result of physical and emotional pressure, and everyone gets fatigued from time to time. If you take too much on, if a lot is happening at home or at work, if you are stressed, or if you are regularly kept awake at night, you can easily become tired and lacking energy. Fatigue is also a central feature of depression, it can accompany and follow an infection, and it is common in people with diabetes, heart disease, thyroid problems and a host of other medical conditions. Iron deficiency, for example, is a common cause of fatigue and women can easily become iron-deficient, especially if their periods are heavy or if they are pregnant or breastfeeding.

How can diet help?

One of the best ways to use your diet to fight fatigue is to raise your blood glucose

self-help to become energized

Evaluate your caffeine intake, and experiment with a one- or two-week break from coffee, tea and cola drinks.

Alcohol and nicotine have energy-sapping effects so you should cut down on or avoid them when fatigued.

Eat plenty of carbohydrate-rich foods such as whole-grain bread, beans and pasta that have a low or medium glycaemic index for a gradual and sustained energy boost (see page 29).

To make the best use of the energy provided by carbohydrates, you need to **eat food containing iron, B-group vitamins, vitamin C, zinc, tryptophan, and co-enzyme Q**. Red meat, liver, shellfish, eggs, cashew nuts, soya beans and dried fruit are good sources of iron, while brown rice, lentils, nuts and sunflower seeds supply plenty of B-group vitamins. Fruits and vegetables provide vitamin C, and you will get zinc from eggs, meat, fish and soya products, and co-enzyme Q (CoQ) from spinach and oily fish. Turkey, chicken and other foods rich in tryptophan (see page 13) are good energy boosters, as are lecithin granules.

Instead of three large meals a day, **try eating several small meals or snacks** throughout the day, and don't eat a large meal less than four hours before bedtime.

levels by eating plenty of energy-boosting foods. However, these should be foods with a low or medium glycaemic index (see page 28), which provide a gradual and sustained release of energy. This is much better than eating sugary or fatty foods with a high glycaemic index, which give a rapid but short-lived boost to your blood glucose levels. For some people, the benefits of foods with a low or medium glycaemic index are enhanced by eating several small meals a day, rather than the traditional three large ones. This reduces the energy-sapping drops in blood glucose levels that happen when there are large gaps between meals, and helps you to avoid the sleepiness that often follows a heavy meal.

These meals should include foods rich in the iron, vitamins, and other nutrients that help your brain and body to use the energy from the carbohydrates.

Although caffeine provides a brief boost of energy and alertness, it can make fatigue worse in the longer term. It also has the potential to be addictive—with energy-sapping withdrawal symptoms—and can increase levels of anxiety and tension.

Chronic Fatigue Syndrome

Sometimes, fatigue can be severe and prolonged, lasting for months or even years and interfering so badly with your ability to function normally that it becomes a condition called Chronic Fatigue Syndrome (CFS).

The term "Chronic Fatigue Syndrome" is a more a description than a diagnosis because we don't know exactly what causes the condition, which is often associated with a number of different illnesses including fibromyalgia, myalgic encephalomyelitis, and irritable bowel syndrome. It is unlikely that there is only one cause of CFS, and none has yet been conclusively identified after many years' intensive research.

The current mainstay of treatment for CFS is a gradual increase in levels of activity, with the patient neither attempting too much when feeling comparatively energetic, nor too little when fatigued.

symptoms of...
CHRONIC FATIGUE SYNDROME

- poor concentration
- poor memory
- aching muscles
- tender glands
- sore throat
- joint pain
- more headaches than usual
- un-refreshing sleep
- fatigue after mild exertion

Diet and CFS

There have been many attempts to treat CFS with food supplements or special diets, but so far the only promising results have been with fish oils and magnesium supplements. So eating plenty of oily fish, such as salmon, and magnesium-rich foods such as nuts (especially Brazil nuts—also rich in mood-elevating selenium), chickpeas, and wheatgerm may help, especially if the fatigue is comparatively mild to moderate. Chocolate, soft drinks, highly processed foods and caffeine all deplete magnesium, so you should probably avoid them if you have CFS.

Some authorities claim that live-yoghurt drinks (probiotics) containing bacteria such as *Lactobacillus acidophilus* or *Lactobacillus casei immunitas* (see page 93) can help in CFS, probably by boosting the immune system. We suggest that you select a probiotics brand that contains only one strain of bacteria, at a concentration of 1 billion per gram.

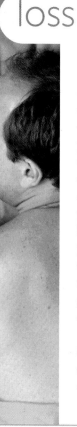

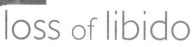

loss of libido

Losing interest in sex is something that can happen to anyone, at any time, and it can be a one-off event, a temporary difficulty, or a more long-lasting problem. Loss of libido can have many causes, both physical and psychological, and although physical illness will very commonly reduce sexual interest, problems with libido are more likely to have a psychological origin. Commonly, people suffering from anxiety, fatigue or depression lose interest in sex while those experiencing mania demonstrate greatly increased sexual interest and very often engage in promiscuous behaviour.

Sexual interest also often falls at times of stress, and when that happens the loss of interest may add to the stress. Stress can be due to work or money worries, or be associated with important events in life such as moving home, changing your job or bereavement. Domestic stress is, unsurprisingly, another common cause of loss of interest, and sometimes one or both partners in a relationship will lose interest in sex (with each other, although perhaps not with other people) because their sex life has become boring.

Problems with sexual performance, which can happen even if desire is undiminished, may be psychological or relationship-based but physical causes are also common. In women, endometriosis may cause sexual problems and be difficult to detect, while many men do not realize that prostate surgery commonly causes failure of erection, as do diabetes, heart and blood vessel disease and neurological disorders.

How can diet help?

Many foods have long been thought to have aphrodisiac properties. For example, carrots and figs earned their aphrodisiac reputations because of their supposed physical resemblance to sexual organs, while shellfish, especially oysters, were thought to produce secretions similar to semen. Unfortunately, very few of these notions are backed up by scientific evidence, but shellfish are great brain foods, rich in essential fatty acids, and oysters also are rich in selenium and zinc. This may or may not enhance sexual prowess, but almost certainly contributes to good mood.

Sunflower seeds and popcorn, that well-known food of love, are rich in the amino acid arginine, which has been claimed to enhance sexual performance. However, the scientific evidence that

STIMULATING SUPPLEMENTS

Many claims have been made for the sexual boosting power of dehydroandrosterone (DHEA), especially in women. This is a natural steroid hormone produced in the adrenal glands, brain and ovaries, and it has been suggested that it can boost low levels of testosterone and increase sex drive. Unfortunately there is no good evidence for this or any of the other alleged beneficial effects of DHEA, and much evidence that it can increase the risk of cancer.

The South American herbal supplements marapuama (*Ptychopetalum olacoides*) and maca (*Lepidium peruvianum*) have long been claimed to stimulate desire and performance in both men and women, and seem to be relatively nontoxic. Yohimbine, which comes from the bark of the West African yohimbe tree (*Corynanthe yohimbe*), is another supplement that has been used in the same way, and is favoured by private clinics for male sexual dysfunction. In such clinics, supplements may be given as creams, which are almost certain to be ineffective unless the patient believes in them.

Eat plenty of shellfish and seafood, which are rich in beneficial vitamins and minerals and are said to improve sexual function and the health of the reproductive system.

Many vitamins, especially B₃ (niacin), B₆ (pyridoxine), C and E, play an important role in sexual function. For both sexes, vitamins B₃ and B₆ help the body to produce its sex hormones, so brown rice, nuts, avocados, almonds, yeast extracts, fish, eggs, meat, sea vegetables and other foods rich in them should be helpful.

If you are lacking in energy, **you may be deficient in trace elements such as iodine, zinc, and iron,** which help your body to utilize the energy you get from your food. Good sources of these nutrients include shellfish and seafood, which are rich in iodine and in zinc (which can also boost levels of testosterone, the male sex hormone), while red meat, liver, eggs and spinach are rich in iron. Spinach also contains co-enzyme Q (CoQ), said to be good for energy and stamina.

For men, **eating foods containing plenty of vitamins C and E** will improve the quality and quantity of semen.

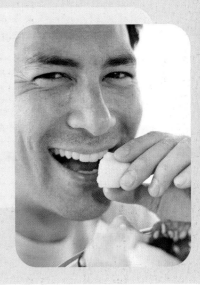

arginine makes any difference is weak, and the effective treatment dose (if there is one) is probably too high to be obtained from food alone. You would need a supplement.

When in doubt...

Do not automatically assume that your problem is psychological. Your first port of call should be to your doctor, who can give you a physical checkup and may order some simple tests that can exclude the common physical causes of sexual problems.

sexual health clinics

There is no need to be embarrassed about discussing sexual problems with your doctor, but some people are, and if you are one of them, you may prefer to visit a private sexual health clinic. If you have a problem and are tempted to try one of these clinics, be cautious. They can be expensive, and although some are very good, others are less reliable and may offer treatments and medications that are of little real value.

hyperactivity and
attention problems

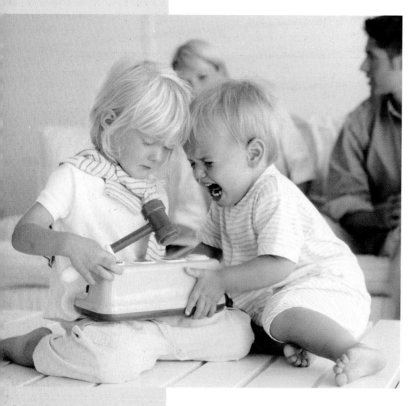

Hyperactivity becomes noticeable about the age of two, when a child becomes increasingly noisy and active. Boys are generally louder and more active.

necessarily having a genetic cause. Some controversial studies in the United States suggest that up to ten percent of children have ADHD, but the National Institute of Mental Health puts the figure at three to five percent. Boys are two to three times more likely to be affected than girls.

Young people with ADHD may have brushes with authority from an early age, both at school and out in the wider world. They may break laws, and become involved with the drug and gang subcultures; as adults, their problems are sometimes not recognized and they risk being written off as bad or personality-disordered people.

Diagnosis and treatment

The diagnosis of ADHD is controversial because it depends entirely on assessing the history of the patient—there are few, if any, objective measurements or tests that can be done. And although inattention, hyperactivity and impulsivity can be measured by psychological testing, the diagnostic tests involved are not truly objective.

The treatment for ADHD is also controversial. For example, medication is widely used to treat it in the United States and is increasingly common in the United Kingdom and Europe, but many people are worried about treating children with powerful drugs, especially where there are some doubts about the accuracy of ADHD diagnoses.

Those who are sceptical about drug use prefer an educational approach, perhaps with individual remedial training

Children are prone to many learning and behavioural problems, but fortunately few of them amount to a full-blown psychiatric disorder such as Attention Deficit Hyperactivity Disorder (ADHD). Children with this disorder suffer from problems such as an inability to concentrate, hyperactive and impulsive behaviour, and aggression.

ADHD is the most common psychiatric disorder in children, but it can also occur (commonly, some say) in adults. There is some evidence that it runs in families, but because it is very common anyway, it may well occur more than once in larger families without because some children can't work effectively within a class but will respond to individual treatment.

The same sceptics also are concerned that the medication used may have potentially serious side effects, its long-term effectiveness is unproven, and that it may increase the risk of drug addiction in the future.

This sceptical approach has merit, but there is plenty of evidence that medication has made a dramatic improvement to children who had previously been entirely unmanageable, deeply unhappy, and falling far short of their personal and educational potential. However, these drugs should be prescribed only by specialists, and their use should be kept under constant review and continued only if they work.

How can diet help?

An improved diet seems to help with ADHD and other behaviour problems in two main ways—by adding beneficial nutrients such as vitamins and minerals, and by subtracting harmful chemicals such as food additives.

The value of adding beneficial nutrients was demonstrated in an important recent study conducted with young offenders in a penal institution in the United Kingdom. Two groups of offenders were selected at random, and one was given nutrient supplements and the other a dummy treatment (placebo). During the study, the prisoners taking the nutrients were involved in nearly

The hyperactive child's general behaviour is similar to his peers but so amplified that it appears much worse. Some doctors, therefore, believe that it is just one end of the normal spectrum of behaviour.

symptoms of...
ADHD

A child, adolescent, or adult may be suffering from ADHD if he or she consistently shows certain characteristic behaviours—inattention, hyperactivity and impulsivity—over a period of time. The condition comes on before the age of seven and the symptoms carry over from school to home, or work to home. If the sufferer is aggressive or rides roughly over the rights of others, his or her behaviour may amount to conduct disorder.

Signs of persistent inattention include an inability to concentrate on work or play, to follow through instructions, to organize, and to persevere, and a tendency to lose things. Hyperactivity and impulsivity are shown by fidgeting, distractibility, inability to keep sitting, restlessness and being ceaselessly full of energy and very talkative. Sometimes, people with ADHD may also suffer from other conditions such as clumsiness (dyspraxia) or reading difficulties (dyslexia).

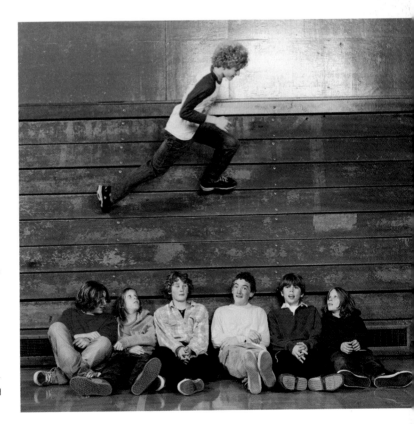

ADHD research

Over the past three decades or so, most of the research into the effects of diet on ADHD has been carried out on young people (almost always young men) confined in penal institutions. During this research, the effects of changing the diet of the research subjects has been measured in terms of changes in behaviour, obedience to rules, number of violent incidents, and so on.

There are problems with interpreting the results in these settings. It may be, for example, that a young person taking part in such a study receives attention from an interested, caring adult, perhaps for the first time in his life, and this in itself may improve behaviour. Moreover, the rules of penal institutions are not necessarily the rules of life outside. An institution provides a constant, regulated environment, and what influences behaviour there is not necessarily what influences it outside. So people are sometimes doubtful about the true value of such research, but that does not detract from its potential importance or its consistent message over the years, which is that improving diet can improve behaviour.

COMMON DRUGS FOR ADHD

CENTRAL NERVOUS SYSTEM STIMULANTS
- methylphenidate
  (short-acting — Ritalin;
  longer-acting — Concerta)
- dextroamphetamine (Dexedrine)

SELECTIVE NORADRENALINE REUPTAKE INHIBITOR, SNRI
- atomoxetine (Strattera)

40 percent fewer violent incidents than the group taking the placebo, but their levels of violence returned to normal once the study was over and they were no longer getting the extra nutrients.

The nutrient supplements that produced this dramatic improvement in behaviour contained vitamins B, C, D and E in doses more or less equivalent to the recommended levels for a normal, healthy diet, except that there was double the usual amount of folic acid. They also contained minerals, again at recommended levels but with higher amounts of chromium and molybdenum, plus omega 3 and omega 6 fatty acids.

We do not know quite why this diet should work, but there are some possible reasons. For example, folic acid aids the metabolism of neurotransmitters such as serotonin (see page 12), and so can help combat depression. Chromium can help in depression, too. In the form of chromium picolinate, it can enhance the absorption of tryptophan and so boost levels of serotonin in the brain.

Why molybdenum should help, we do not know. This mineral is present in the body in trace amounts only, so deficiency is most unlikely. It is known to be important for the metabolism of most nutrients, as well as being necessary for strong teeth, but its role in behaviour is entirely unknown. As for fatty acids, there seems little doubt of their importance in the normal working of the brain (see page 24) and they appear to help in depression and other disorders. Taking probiotics (see page 92) and adopting a high-protein diet also may be helpful.

What to avoid

The second beneficial way in which you can alter the diet of a child (or adult) with ADHD is by cutting out foods

Avoid serving your child ready-prepared meals, packaged food or foods and drinks that are high in additives. Commercially produced fish fingers, burgers, chicken nuggets, processed cheese slices, sausages, carbonated drinks, cakes and biscuits should be off the menu.

Supplements—Omega 3 and Omega 6 fatty acids have been shown to improve the behaviour of children with ADHD. Since many children won't eat fish, your best bet is to give them a fish-oil or plant-based supplement.

Increase your child's intake of vitamin B_1 (thiamine) and B_6 found in potatoes, whole grains, nuts, seeds, eggs and meat.

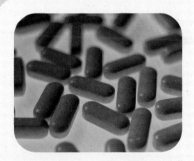

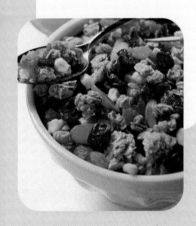

Zinc, calcium and magnesium are minerals important for improving concentration. If your child is not eating enough dairy products, whole grains or green leafy vegetables, consider introducing a supplement.

Ensure that your child **eats carbohydrate foods at the same time as some protein food**. The carbohydrates will allow the tryptophan in the protein food to be taken up more effectively by the brain to be subsequently turned into serotonin.

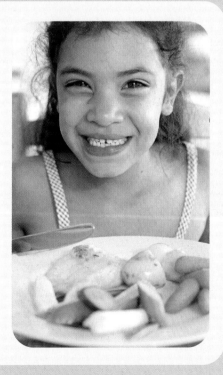

containing additives thought to trigger behaviour problems, and foods associated with allergies.

The food colouring tartrazine yellow, for example, has been implicated consistently with hyperactivity in children, which it probably causes by reducing levels of essential trace minerals such as zinc. The Feingold Diet, developed in the United States in the 1960s to help hyperactive children, involves eliminating this and other petroleum-based artificial food dyes, flavourings and preservatives (see box, opposite). Additives can affect normally active children too, and crankiness and restlessness in a young child may often follow the consumption of brightly coloured sweets or drinks.

The diet also eliminates foods rich in salicylates, including ketchup and many otherwise nutritious foods such as nuts and some dried and fresh fruits. But the evidence that salicylates play a significant part in hyperactivity is less strong than that for food additives, except in children who are sensitive to aspirin (salicylic acid), so the elimination of additives is probably a better and more practical course. However, aspirin itself should not be given to children, because of a rare but often fatal side effect known as Reye's syndrome.

ALLERGIES AND INTOLERANCE

Food allergies have long been associated with hyperactivity and many other health problems. A true allergy involves an over-strong reaction of the immune system, with the release of chemicals (especially histamine) that cause unpleasant symptoms such as rashes.

The simplest symptom of a food allergy is an increased pulse rate. You can test your child's reaction to a given food by first establishing his or her normal, "baseline" pulse rate, then seeing if the rate increases about half an hour after your child eats the food, the time it takes to absorb it. If the pulse rate increases by 10 percent or more (normal is around 70 to 80 beats a minute), there is a chance your child may be allergic to, or intolerant of, the food in question.

A food intolerance is similar to a food allergy but it need not involve the immune system, and examples include intolerance to lactose (milk sugar) or food additives. Food aversions reflect personal dislike of the food concerned, where symptoms occur only if someone knows (or believes) that he or she has eaten the food concerned.

You can boost your child's immune system, and perhaps reduce the effects of food allergies or intolerance, with probiotics, quercitin (contained in onions and garlic, and available in supplements) and foods rich in B-group vitamins.

It's quite common for children to develop aversions to certain colours, flavours, or types of foods. These dislikes are usually transient, however, and may be overcome simply with more "kid-pleasing" ways of serving food.

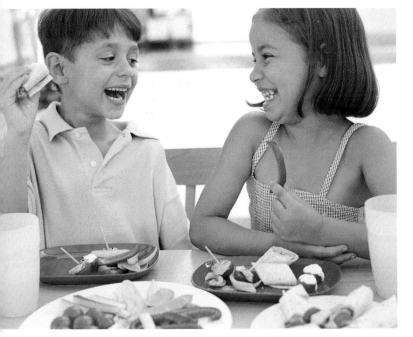

food additives to avoid

There is strong evidence that cutting out manufactured foods containing certain synthetic additives can reduce the symptoms of ADHD. It is good practice, therefore, to always check the labels of foods before you buy them to see if any of the substances listed below are included in the list of ingredients.

SUBSTANCE	US CODE	EU CODE	BANNED IN
COLOURINGS			
Tartrazine	FD&C Yellow No.5	E102	Austria, Norway
Quinoline Yellow	FD&C Yellow No.10	E104	USA, Australia, Norway
Yellow 7G		E107	USA, Australia
Sunset Yellow FCF, Orange Yellow S	FD&C Yellow No.6	E110	Norway
Cochineal, Carminic acid, Carmines		E120	
Azorubine, Carmoisine		E122	USA, Austria, Norway, Sweden
Amaranth	FD&C Red No.2	E123	USA, Austria, Norway, Russia, and other countries
Ponceau 4R, Cochineal Red A	FD&C Red No.4	E124	USA, Norway
Erythrosine	FD&C Red No.3	E127	USA, Norway
Red 2G		E128	Australia and many other countries except United Kingdom
Indigotine, Indigo Carmine	FD&C Blue No.2	E132	Norway
Brilliant Blue FCF	FD&C Blue Dye No.1	E133	Austria, Belgium, France, Germany, Norway, Sweden, Switzerland
Caramel (colouring)		E150a, b, c, d	
Brilliant Black BN, Black PN		E151	USA, Australia, Austria, Belgium, Denmark, France, Germany, Norway, Sweden, Switzerland
Brown FK		E154	USA
Brown HT		E155	USA, Austria, Belgium, Denmark, France, Germany, Norway, Sweden, Switzerland
Annatto, arnatto, bixin, norbixin		E160b	
PRESERVATIVES			
Benzoic acid		E210	
Sodium benzoate		E211	
Sulphur dioxide		E220	
Sodium nitrite		E250	
Sodium nitrate		E251	
ANTIOXIDANTS			
Tertiary butyl hydroquinone (TBHQ)		E319	
Butylated hydroxyanisole (BHA)		E320	Japan
Butylated hydroxytoluene (BHT)		E321	Japan

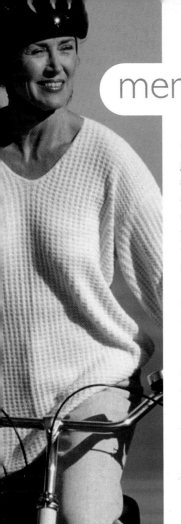

memory problems

One of the more frustrating aspects of growing older is that your memory slowly but steadily declines, starting at around the age of twenty. This decline is a gradual process that causes few real problems, and the vast majority of people who worry that they may be losing their memories are usually mistaken.

What many people assume to be memory loss is often simply the result of poor concentration. This can happen either because you are not interested in what you are doing, or because your ability to concentrate is diminished, for example by worry, depression, thinking about something else, a physical illness, or a hormone imbalance. There is almost certainly little if anything physically wrong with your memory, which will return to normal when the underlying cause is resolved.

However, memory problems that do have a physical cause will get worse. This can be a steady and progressive decline or can occur in steps, with intervals of apparent normality in between. Much more often than not, it is other people who notice a problem, and the person affected will be unaware of it. Any medical assessment of memory problems must include a full physical checkup, as well as a full appraisal of what else is going on in the person's life at that time.

Slowing the decline

While you can't halt the normal decline in memory that comes with age, you can help to keep your memory working as well as it can. Keeping yourself physically active with regular exercise improves your circulation, which helps your blood to deliver energy and oxygen to your brain, and makes you more alert and able to concentrate. If you keep mentally active, your brain will respond by creating new connections between its cells to help it store and retrieve information more easily.

How can diet help?

A balanced diet with adequate amounts of vitamins will contribute to your general health, while particular foods—such as fish—also may help both memory and some of the common underlying physical causes of memory problems, such as poor circulation of blood in the brain.

Fish has not been called an ideal brain food for nothing. The omega 3 fatty acids that it contains, especially docosahexanoic acid (DHA) and eicosapentanoic acid (EPA), seem most important for a healthy brain and a good memory. They also appear to be essential to the health of the heart and blood vessels.

Studies have shown that older people who are low in DHA are nearly twice as likely as those high in DHA to develop dementia, the chronic mental confusion that afflicts some elderly people and makes it hard or impossible for them to lead normal lives. Salmon is particularly rich in DHA and EPA, but other cold-water oily fish such as tuna, mackerel and sardines are also excellent sources. Many other foods contain different fatty acids that the body can convert into DHA and EPA. These foods include flaxseed, avocados, nuts and shiso (also called perilla or Japanese basil) and other green vegetables. Their fatty acid content is not as great as that of fish, and not everyone is able to convert these fatty acids to DHA and EPA, but they form a valuable addition to the diet.

The neurotransmitter acetylcholine, which the brain makes from a substance called choline, also appears to be important for a good memory. Evidence that eating foods rich in choline and phosphatidylcholine (the main source of choline), such as eggs, beef, liver and soya products, can help to improve memory is scanty, but it won't do you any harm. A small number of people, perhaps no more than one in 1000, may have difficulty metabolizing choline, and may be unfortunate enough to smell strongly of fish if they take extra amounts of it. This side effect is not dangerous, but is undoubtedly unpleasant.

Antioxidants, found in various foods but especially in fruit and vegetables, seem to play a vital role in protecting the brain from damage by free radicals, which are natural but potentially harmful by-products of cell metabolism. So it is essential not to restrict your consumption of fruit and vegetables, even if you are following a low-carbohydrate, high-protein weight-loss diet.

Herbal products

Many products on the market claim to boost memory and brain function, but the hype outweighs the reality in almost every case. Of all these products, ginkgo (*Ginkgo biloba*) and phosphatidyl serine (PS) have the most evidence in their favour, but even that is inconclusive. Other compounds, such as co-enzyme Q, acetyl L-carnitine, and Siberian ginseng (*Eleutherococcus senticosus*) have their proponents, but the evidence for their benefits is scanty, or not based on research on humans. Their side effects are few, but there can be a possibly harmful interaction between ginkgo and anticoagulant drugs such as warfarin.

Keep physically and mentally active.
Do aerobic exercise at least three times a week and keep your brain ticking over by doing puzzles or setting yourself a new task to learn.

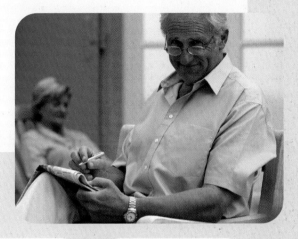

Cut down on alcohol consumption: excess alcohol hinders concentration and interferes with the brain's ability to store and retrieve information.

Supplements: Omega-3-rich fish oils are recommended as is lecithin, a good source of choline. It is available as a food supplement in granule form, useful for sprinkling over cereals and salads.

Herbs Ginkgo (*Ginkgo biloba*) is said to have some effect.

Eating oily fish at least twice a week provides good protection for the brain.

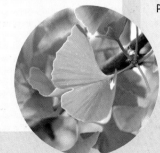

bipolar disorder and schizophrenia

Bipolar disorder and schizophrenia are common mental disorders, each affecting about one percent of the population. Both are potentially disabling, and require professional diagnosis and treatment, but with proper medication most sufferers are able to lead reasonably normal lives.

What is bipolar disorder?

Also called bipolar affective disorder or manic depression, it comes in two main varieties and several sub-varieties. Bipolar I disorder is "classic" manic depression, where people suffer recurring bouts of clinical depression and mania (a highly euphoric state of mental and physical hyperactivity). They may, over the years, suffer more from one than the other—most people have recurrent depression more often than recurrent mania—but they clearly have both. People with bipolar II disorder experience recurrent clinical depression, but they have a history of at least one episode of feeling high that falls short of clinical mania. This

distinction matters, because the treatment of bipolar disorder differs from that of "pure" depression, even if recurrent.

How can diet help?

There is some evidence that omega 3 fish oils can be helpful, and other beneficial foods include nuts and seeds (especially peanuts and pumpkin seeds) and whole-grain fibres rich in magnesium, the calming mineral. Reducing tyrosine levels (see page 16) can treat mania. If you have been prescribed a medication, keep on taking it as instructed. If you are on lithium, which sometimes can affect the function of the thyroid gland, eating Brazil nuts and other foods rich in selenium can improve your thyroid function. You also need to drink sufficient water to balance the lithium levels.

COMMON DRUGS

BIPOLAR DISORDER
- lithium (Eskalith, Lithane, Lithobid)
- valproic acid or divalproex sodium (Depakote)
- lamotrigine (Lamictal)
- carbamazepine (Tegretol)
- olanzapine (Zyprexa)
- risperidone (Risperdal)

SCHIZOPHRENIA
- aripiprazole (Abilify)
- clozapine (Clozaril)
- olanzapine (Zyprexa)
- quetiapine (Seroquel)
- risperidone (Risperdal)
- ziprasidone (Geodon)

the sodium-potassium connection

We do not know the precise cause of bipolar disorder, but it probably involves the movement of sodium and potassium within the brain's neurons (see page 10), and an imbalance of the main neurotransmitters dopamine, serotonin and noradrenaline. Lithium, one of the mainstays of the treatment of bipolar disorder, is similar to sodium and it reduces the neurons' production of inositol (see page 28), an important sugar-like molecule that helps with the transmission of brain signals. Reduced levels of inositol seem to lower mood, hence the use of inositol supplements or inositol-rich foods in the treatment of depression.

Eat plenty of foods containing omega 3 essential fatty acids such as oily fish, particularly salmon and mackerel.

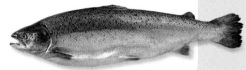

Reduce or cut out tyrosine-rich foods such as mature cheeses, beans, chicken, cured meats, liver, pickled vegetables, chocolate, aubergines, potatoes, spinach and tomatoes during periods of mania.

Avoid alcohol and caffeine, and resist the temptation to use cannabis to relax, as it is likely to make your symptoms worse.

If you are taking lithium, **drink plenty of water**, particularly in warm weather. Kidney function decreases when it is hot, preventing lithium from being excreted in the urine.

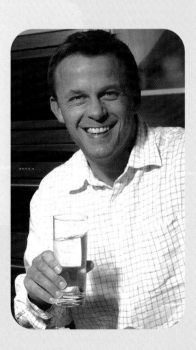

schizophrenia

Schizophrenia is a severe mental disorder, and people suffering from it often experience frightening symptoms such as hearing voices inside their heads, or believing that other people are controlling their minds. Its causes are complex. A common feature of the illness is an imbalance of some of the normal brain chemicals, especially dopamine. This disordered brain chemistry is the target of the drugs used to treat the condition.

HOW CAN DIET HELP?
People with schizophrenia often have poor physical as well as mental health, because they often live chaotically. They may rely on sugary convenience or fast foods which increase the chances of heart disease and diabetes. Eating a good diet will improve their physical health and, together with proper medication, can improve their overall condition.

Compounds such as alpha lipoic acid, found in spinach and broccoli, can help to reduce heart-damaging cholesterol levels and control diabetes, while foods with a medium or low glycaemic index (see page 28) can help improve the mood by preventing rapid fluctuations of glucose levels in the blood. Caffeine intake should be reduced and preferably avoided altogether. And because overactivity of dopamine is at least part of the problem in schizophrenia, it may be worth cutting down on dopamine-rich foods such as meat. People with schizophrenia may benefit particularly from a vegetarian diet.

Foods rich in omega 3 and omega 6 fatty acids also can be beneficial and, although this view is not held by mainstream psychiatrists, vitamin B_3 (niacin) is also recommended because it aids the proper function of other neurotransmitters, especially serotonin. Good sources include cereals, peanut butter, potatoes baked in their skins, long-grain brown rice and whole-wheat bread.

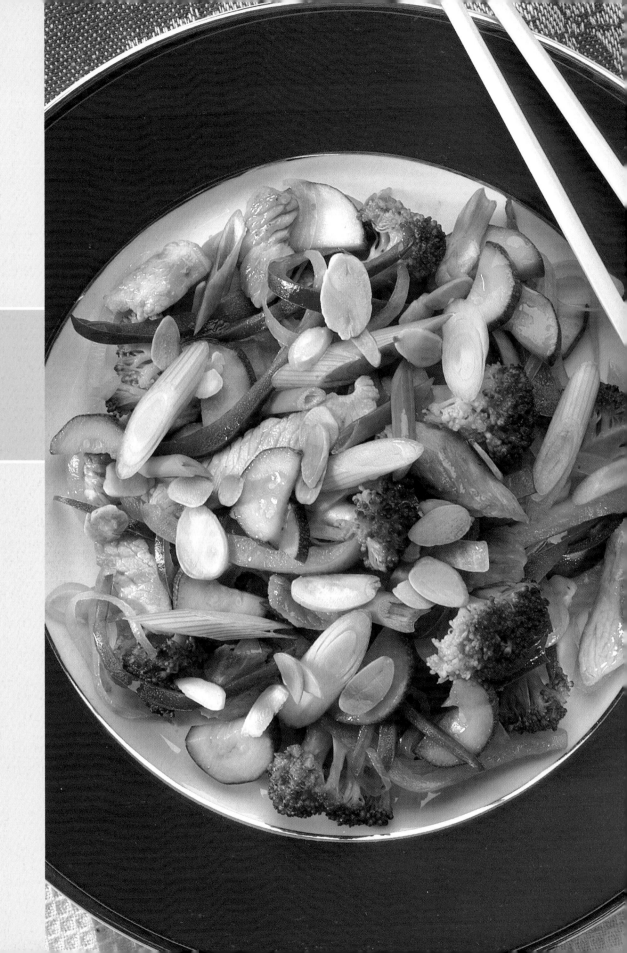

5

IMPROVING NUTRIENT VALUE

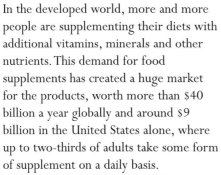

food supplements added extras

In the developed world, more and more people are supplementing their diets with additional vitamins, minerals and other nutrients. This demand for food supplements has created a huge market for the products, worth more than $40 billion a year globally and around $9 billion in the United States alone, where up to two-thirds of adults take some form of supplement on a daily basis.

Many people who take supplements do so because they genuinely need them. These include pregnant women (who need vitamin B$_{12}$ and folate supplements, and may need iron supplements); older people, who may not eat properly; and some people who follow particular diets. For example, a strict vegan diet can be low in the essential nutrients found in meat, so a strict vegan may need to take supplements to achieve a fully balanced diet. But most nutritionists believe that the majority of people eating balanced diets have little need for supplements.

Apart from being appropriate only in special cases, some supplements can actually be harmful if you take too much of them. An important example is iron, which is necessary for life because it forms the core of haemoglobin. This substance makes our blood red and allows red blood cells to deliver the oxygen that our body and brain cells need to function and survive. People who have anaemia—a low level of haemoglobin in the blood—need extra iron in their diets, but most people get all they need from their food. Too much iron can be dangerous, especially for children, as an excess can have serious consequences ranging from liver damage to death.

Many food supplements are less toxic than iron, because the body will simply use the amount that it needs and discard any excess. However, taking too much of most minerals can have toxic effects, and some vitamins can be harmful in large doses. For example, vitamin C seems safe enough, but an overdose of vitamin A can cause blindness and even death.

Should you take supplements?

In theory, a healthy, balanced diet will contain all the nutrients you need, but some people argue that modern farming methods and food processing have reduced the nourishment available from food. This seems like common sense, but it is highly controversial because there seems to be no clear evidence based on direct comparison with the food produced in the past, so the jury is still out.

In this book, we assume the normal diet to be one that incorporates a balance of nutrients and contains fat, fibre, protein, vitamins and minerals in proportions that can be best used by the body. We suggest modifications only where there is evidence that these can have a positive effect on mental health.

coenzyme q

Coenzyme Q (CoQ) is not a vitamin, but its functions are similar. It seems to be essential to the way that cells use energy, and works as an antioxidant—it helps to mop up potentially harmful oxygen-containing compounds called free radicals, which are by-products of cell metabolism. CoQ is believed to boost the immune system, and has been suggested as an extra treatment for Alzheimer's disease.

Supplements and mental health

In general, food supplements may be beneficial to your mental health when your diet is lacking in certain nutrients, not because there is anything to be gained by taking more of them than your body needs. Making up for deficiencies is often the key to good mental health.

For example, deficiencies of the B vitamins (such as B_1, B_3, B_6, B_{12} and folic acid) are all associated with concentration problems, depressed mood, and even psychosis. In alcoholics and other people who are grossly malnourished, deficiency of vitamin B_1 (thiamine) can have major effects on the brain, and plays an important part in the potentially fatal brain condition called Wernicke's encephalopathy. People with this condition suffer confusion or delirium, paralysed eye muscles, and difficulty in walking. Deficiency of vitamin B_3 (niacin) causes pellagra, a nutritional disease that has mental illness as one of its major symptoms.

The B vitamins also act as essential cofactors, substances that allow important enzymes in the body to operate properly. Vitamins B_6, B_{12} and folic acid are essential in this, and folic acid in particular appears to be important in the successful development of the nervous system. This is why folic acid supplements are often given to pregnant women, especially those who otherwise might be at risk of having babies with conditions such as spina bifida.

Deficiencies of the minerals calcium and magnesium also appear to play an important part in psychiatric disorders. As with other nutrients, the evidence that deficiencies of these minerals has a harmful effect is much stronger than the evidence that taking more of them than you actually need has a beneficial effect.

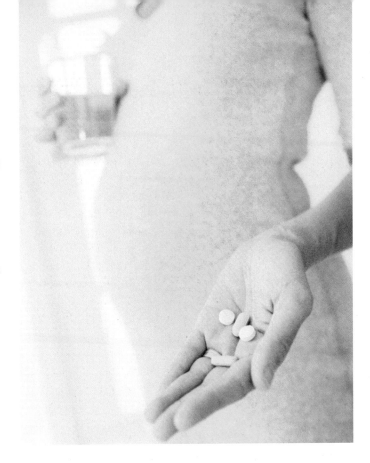

This is even more true of the so-called trace elements, vital compounds that are present in very small quantities in the body. For example, many people are deficient in zinc, which is an essential cofactor with many enzymes. Serious zinc deficiency has been associated with a range of mental illnesses, but the benefits of taking extra zinc have not been established by rigorous clinical trials.

This is also the case with selenium, another enzyme cofactor, although some interesting studies have indicated an overall improvement in general mood and psychiatric "wellness" in people who regularly supplement their diets with it, so it may be worth trying. Brazil nuts are particularly rich in selenium, so that two or three Brazil nuts a day would make up the lack of selenium that is common in the Western diet.

A healthy balanced diet should contain all the nutrients you need, but there may be times—such as during pregnancy or in later life—when a supplement could prove beneficial.

probiotics

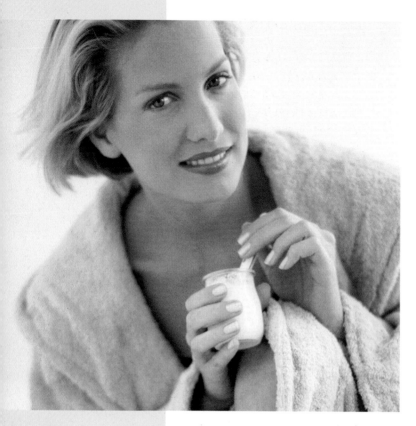

An important but often overlooked contribution to your health and sense of wellbeing comes from your intestines, which complete the process of digestion that begins in your stomach. Your intestines break down the partly digested food that comes from your stomach, separate out the nutrients it contains, and absorb them for use by your body and brain.

When your intestines are not working efficiently, you may not get the full benefit of some of the nutrients in your food, no matter how healthy your diet is. If these nutrients are among those important for your mental health, then having a disordered digestion can often bring unsettled emotions. One way to help keep your intestines healthy is to eat foods containing probiotics, which are bacteria that do not cause disease and can have a beneficial effect on your health. They are, in a sense, "living drugs".

The bugs in your body

Your body is home to trillions of bacteria, including around a thousand billion on your skin, ten billion in your mouth, and a hundred trillion in your gastrointestinal tract. The great majority of these bacteria, which weigh a total of about 3 pounds (1.4 kg), are at worst neutral and at best actively helpful to your general wellbeing, and have been called "the body's hidden organ".

Most of the bacteria you carry—some 2.2 pounds (1 kg) of them—live in your intestines where they make up what is known as the normal gut flora. This normal gut flora consists of around 400 different species of bacteria, some of which produce B-group vitamins

antibiotics and probiotics

Life-savers though they are, antibiotics do not discriminate between "good" and "bad" bacteria. They tend to kill them all. So although they benefit you by fighting infections, they can also cause problems by damaging the fragile ecosystem of your gut bacteria. The common experience of feeling tired and "washed out" after a course of antibiotics may be due to loss of the normal gut flora, and the bacteria that recolonize your gut when you stop taking the antibiotics may not be entirely of the beneficial type. So it's a good idea to take probiotics during and after taking a course of antibiotics to help restore the levels of helpful bacteria in your gut and limit the growth of the harmful type.

(including folic acid) and vitamin K, and also help you to digest your food. The aim of foods containing probiotics is to boost the numbers of these helpful bacteria in the gut.

Probiotic foods

Most of the foods that contain probiotics are fermented milk products such as live yoghurts and yoghurt-based supplement drinks. Because yoghurt often contains considerable amounts of sugar, the supplement drinks may be a better source of the billion or so bacteria per millilitre that you need to take three or more times a week (not necessarily every day) for effective cover.

There are several groups of probiotic bacteria used in these products, but the most common are various species of *Lactobacillus* (including *Lactobacillus bulgaricus* and *Lactobacillus acidophilus*) and several species of *Bifidobacterium*. *Lactobacillus acidophilus* is found normally in the small intestine and the vagina. It inhibits the growth of potentially harmful bacteria such as *E. coli* (*Escherichia coli*),

PREBIOTICS

There is some evidence that you can enhance the effect of probiotic foods by also taking supplements containing substances called prebiotics. Prebiotics encourage the growth of probiotic bacteria within the gut and include lactulose, one of a group of sugars called oligosaccharides. Lactulose is commonly used as a food supplement in Japan, but in the United Kingdom it is used on prescription (and as an over-the-counter medicine, Regulose) as a gentle treatment for constipation.

did you know?

The idea that you can improve your health by boosting the numbers of beneficial bacteria in your intestines was first suggested around 1900 by Russian immunologist Ilya Mechnikov (1845–1916), a researcher at the Pasteur Institute in Paris, France. He learned that Bulgarians supposedly had longer lives than people of other countries because they regularly ate yoghurt containing live bacteria, and he suggested that these bacteria protected them from the ageing effect of harmful microbes in their intestines.

and of yeasts such as *Candida albicans*, which causes thrush. It can also enhance the immune system by producing the antiviral compound interferon. *Bifidobacterium* lives more in the large intestine (the colon), where it produces vitamin B, digests lactose (milk sugar), and soaks up excess ammonia released during the process of digestion.

Research has shown that probiotics not only promote gut health but can also help treat a number of complaints including irritable bowel syndrome, food allergies and diarrhoea. For example, *Bifidobacterium* and *Lactobacillus*, especially the strain called LGG (*Lactobacillus rhamnosus* GG), have been used successfully to prevent diarrhoea caused by changes in the gut flora when travelling abroad, and to treat diarrhoea caused by taking antibiotics. *Bifidobacterium* has also been used successfully to treat lactose intolerance and other food allergies, and it may help the body to fight food-poisoning bacteria including the potentially fatal *E. coli* 0157.

raw foods

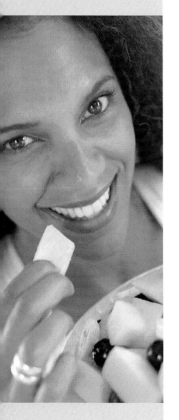

Cooking enhances the taste of many foods—some are virtually inedible unless cooked—but the downside of cooking can be a loss of important nutrients, especially vitamins. So eating foods raw can be more nutritious than eating them cooked, and raw food should have an honoured place in any healthy diet.

We eat raw foods rather more than we may think. Milk, cheese, fruit, salads, and nuts, and many types of cured, smoked and salted meat and fish, are all raw or nearly-raw products. Worries about disease may discourage us from eating raw beef, but the growing Western enjoyment of Japanese cuisine often involves eating fresh, uncooked fish in the form of sushi (raw fish with vinegared rice) and sashimi (thin slices of raw fish). As long as raw food is fresh, and prepared with scrupulous hygiene, there is normally little or no health risk in eating it.

Preserving nutrients

Avoid peeling vegetables as many of the nutrients and the essential fibre are found just under the skin. Instead, scrub the skin with a vegetable brush under running cold water. Wash them just before eating to protect against vitamin loss. Think before discarding broccoli and cauliflower stalks, as these are rich in vitamins. If possible, don't cut fruit and vegetables into small pieces as this exposes more of the surface to the air and nutrients will be dispersed.

Fabulous fruit

Thanks to refrigeration, airfreight, and global trading, we now have easy access to a wider range of fruit than ever before, and the availability of different types of fruit no longer depends on the local growing seasons. As food, fruits have a lot going for them—they are tasty, healthy, and need little or no preparation, they can be served in a variety of appetizing ways, and fruit juices (see page 96) are a healthy alternative to soft drinks.

Raw fruits contain vitamins and minerals that help both body and brain to function properly. For example, most are rich in vitamin C, and apricots, papaya, melons and mangoes contain good amounts of betacarotene, which the body converts into vitamin A. Both vitamin C and vitamin A are powerful antioxidants that help protect brain and body cells from damage by free radicals, natural but harmful by-products of cell activity. Most fruits supply useful amounts of folic acid and of dietary fibre, which aids bowel function and reduces cholesterol, and dried apricots, dried figs and prunes are good sources of iron and calcium.

Salad spectacular

Green, leafy vegetables range from lettuce and watercress, which are eaten raw, to the more robust cabbage, spinach and broccoli. The latter are usually cooked, but they can be even tastier and more nutritious when served raw in salads. Leafy vegetables are great sources of betacarotene, vitamin C, folic acid and dietary fibre, and a bowl of salad is quite bulky and filling yet very low in calories. Because salad vegetables are rich in antioxidants, they can be the corner-stone of a detoxing diet that boosts energy and vitality (see page 100).

Salad dressings can transform even the blandest leaves into something special, but while the calorie content of simple oil-

and-vinegar dressings is small you might want to go easy on full-fat dressings if you are watching your weight.

Another good way to liven up a green salad is to add tasty and colourful carrots, tomatoes and peppers. These are good sources of betacarotene and vitamin C, and tomatoes also contain the antioxidant lycopene.

Slimming snacks

Raw fruit and vegetables make ideal snacks between meals because they are healthy, nonfattening, and don't rot your teeth. And if you have young children, you can inculcate an early love of raw food by getting them into the habit of snacking on fruit or vegetables instead of sweets, biscuits or crisps.

A tasty way to eat raw vegetables is to cut them into sticks (crudités) and to serve them with a savoury dip made of low-fat yoghurt. Alternatively, substitute pieces of fruit for the vegetables and eat them with a sweet dip.

In the ancient world, lettuce was thought to reduce sexual desire and performance. However the Romans believed that rocket was a powerful aphrodisiac that could neutralize lettuce's passion-killing effects.

healthy fruits and vegetables

	VITAMIN A*	VITAMIN C	VITAMIN E	DIETARY FIBRE	CALCIUM	IRON	FOLIC ACID
FRUIT							
oranges		●●●		●			●
grapefruit		●●●		●			●
strawberries		●●●					●
raspberries		●●●		●●			●
apricots:							
fresh	●	●			●	●	
canned	●●	●●			●	●	
dried	●●●	●●●		●	●●●	●●●	
bananas		●●		●			●
papaya	●●●	●●●		●			
VEGETABLES							
carrots	●●●	●		●●			
broccoli	●●●	●●●	●	●		●	●●
cabbage	●●	●●		●			●
spinach	●●●	●	●	●●		●●	●●●
peppers:							
red	●●●	●●●					
green	●	●●●					
tomatoes	●●●	●●	●				
avocados	●		●	●			●

The fruits and vegetables in this table are examples of good sources of important vitamins and minerals—the more circles, the higher the nutrient content. *As betacarotene.

fruit and vegetable juices

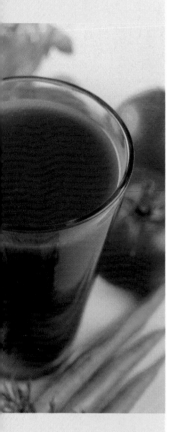

Drinking juices is a good way to boost your intake of the vitamins, minerals and other beneficial ingredients of fruits and vegetables. And because juices are easy to digest, your body can quickly assimilate and use all these health-giving nutrients.

Supermarkets and stores stock a wide range of fruit and vegetable juices in cans, cartons and bottles. Many are excellent, but you should always check the labels carefully if you want to avoid products that are heavily diluted with water or contain sweeteners, flavourings, colourings and other additives.

Ready-prepared juices are convenient to buy and store and need little or no preparation, but the freshest and possibly most nutritious and tasty juices are those you make yourself from fresh fruit or vegetables. Making your own juices is an easy process, but the method to use will depend on the type of fruit or vegetable you are juicing.

Fruit juices

To get the juice from an orange or other citrus fruit, you can simply cut it in half and squeeze it or use a manual extractor or press. But for most other fruits and for vegetables (and if you want to prepare large quantities of juice) you need an electric juicing machine or a food processor with a juicer attachment. These machines quickly reduce the fruit or vegetables to a pulp and squeeze the juice out of them. But whichever extraction method you use, some of the nutrient content (and most of the dietary fibre) is inevitably left behind in the pulp, so drinking juices is not a substitute for eating fruit and vegetables. No matter how much fresh juice you drink, it only

KEEP IT CLEAN

Always clean fruit or vegetables thoroughly before juicing them, because any dirt or bacteria on their surfaces will get into the juice when you extract it. You should also carefully cut away and discard any bruised or damaged areas, because these can harbour dangerous bacteria. As an extra precaution, don't give fresh fruit or vegetable juices to young children, the elderly, or someone with a weakened immune system. Instead, buy them juices that are clearly labelled as pasteurized (pasteurization is a heat treatment that kills harmful bacteria).

counts as one portion of the five daily helpings of fruit and vegetables recommended by nutritionists.

Fruit juices are rich in vitamins, especially the antioxidants vitamin C and betacarotene (a source of vitamin A), and in folic acid and minerals such as calcium, potassium and magnesium. They also provide energy, in the form of fructose (fruit sugar). The most popular fruit juices include orange, grapefruit, lemon, apple and grape. Sometimes juice may need sweetening, but make sure you add just enough sugar or sugar substitute to make the juice pleasantly drinkable.

The juices of many other fruits, such as berry fruits, peaches, apricots, mangoes and pineapple, are often either too intensely flavoured, too sweet, or too bitter to be drunk on their own. The best way to make them drinkable is to mix them with apple juice or grape juice, or make them into smoothies by blending them with, for example, bananas and yoghurt (use an electric blender for this).

Vegetable juices

Most people appreciate the value of fruit juices, but fewer realize that juices from vegetables can be just as nutritious. For example, while apricot, mango, and citrus fruit juices are rich in vitamin A and betacarotene, the juices of many vegetables including carrot, spinach and watercress are also rich sources of this compound. Tangerine and kale juices are both rich in vitamin B_1 (thiamine), cherry and kale juices in vitamin B_2, citrus fruit and kale juices (again) in vitamin B_3, and melon juice and juice from Brussels sprouts contain lots of folic acid. Citrus and watercress juices are both particularly rich in vitamin C.

Vegetable juices often taste better when you mix them, either with other vegetable juices or with fruit juices, and you should not be afraid to experiment.

FRUIT JUICE AND DIABETES

If you suffer from diabetes, remember that fruit juices contain sugar and drinking too much of them might be hazardous for you.

For instance, a blend of fennel, parsley, spinach, and cucumber juices tastes great, is rich in vitamins and minerals (including iron), and is an excellent energy booster. If you want a calming drink rather than one that lifts your energy, try a cocktail of juices rich in B-vitamins and calcium, such as watercress, kale and carrots.

Other juice combinations worth trying include carrot and apple; tomato and celery; beet, carrot and tomato; and avocado, apple and banana. It is best to drink mixed juices as soon after preparing them as possible, because the different components of the mixture start to separate quite quickly.

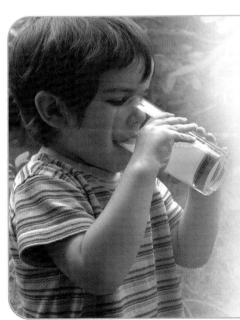

JUICES FOR CHILDREN

Pure juices can be a healthy part of a child's diet, but there are limits to how much juice a child should drink each day because too much can lead to stomach problems, diarrhoea and tooth decay. To avoid such problems:

- juices should not be given to infants under 6 months old
- infants over 6 months old should not get juice from feeding bottles or spouted cups that allow them to drink juice easily throughout the day
- infants should not get juice at bedtime
- for children aged 1 to 6, intake of juice should be limited to 125 to 175 ml (4 to 6 ounces) per day
- for children aged 7 to 18, juice intake should be between 240 to 360 ml (8 and 12 ounces) per day
- children should be encouraged to eat whole fruits and vegetables

sea vegetables

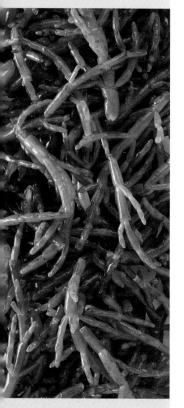

Sea vegetables are wild foods growing along the coasts or in the sea, and include samphire, salicornia, and edible seaweeds. They are something of an acquired taste for most people, but they are good brain foods because they are rich in vitamins and minerals.

Samphire (*Crithmum maritimum*), also called rock samphire, is a small European shrub with long, fleshy leaves and a noticeably salty flavour. It can be boiled or steamed and eaten like asparagus, or as an accompaniment to meat or seafood.

Salicornia (*Salicornia bigelovii*), the North American equivalent of rock samphire, has spiky green leaves and looks a little like a miniature cactus. It is best eaten fresh in salads or as a garnish, as it tends to have a very salty flavour when it is boiled or steamed. Samphire and salicornia both contain good amounts of vitamins A and C, plus minerals such as calcium, iron and magnesium.

> **AGAR**
> Made from several species of red seaweed, agar (or agar-agar) is widely used in the food industry as a thickener and stabilizer. It is also sold in health-food shops, and vegetarians find it useful as an alternative to gelatin (an animal product) for making jellies and desserts.

Seaweeds

Edible seaweeds are rich in valuable nutrients that keep the brain healthy and have many other benefits, including protecting against heart disease and stroke and helping keep the skin in good condition. They are generally about ten times richer in minerals than land vegetables, with particularly high levels of iodine, calcium, potassium, magnesium and iron. Seaweeds are also rich in vitamins A, B (including B_{12}), C, D, E and K, they are a good source of protein, and the number of calories in a serving of seaweed is minimal.

Seaweeds have been an important food in many regions of eastern Asia for thousands of years, but in the West, seaweed has played a much smaller part in people's diets except in some coastal communities. For example, a type of seaweed called laver is eaten in South Wales and southwest England, where it is

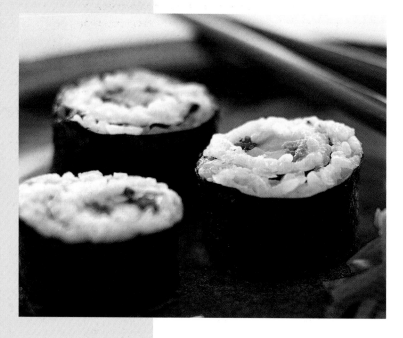

As much as a quarter of all food in the Japanese diet contains some variety of seaweed, used to enhance the flavour of salads, soups and savoury dishes.

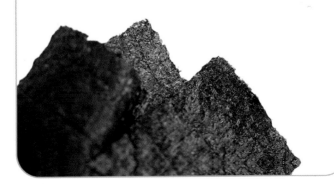

mixed with oatmeal and fried to make the traditional dish known as laver bread, and dulse is a commonly used seaweed along the coasts of Ireland and eastern Canada. Dulse is rich in iron, as well as iodine, phosphorus, potassium, magnesium and vitamins B_6 and B_{12}, and it has a high protein content. It can be shredded and used as a garnish or in salads, or dried and flaked for use as a seasoning or salt replacement. Sun-dried dulse is eaten as a snack in Canada.

But it is the Japanese and Koreans who currently seem to use seaweed the most. Many of the common Japanese seaweeds are easily found in dried form in supermarkets and delicatessens in the West, and sushi is frequently wrapped in thin sheets of a seaweed called nori.

Nori, sold in small sheets, is perhaps the most versatile of the seaweeds because it makes an excellent wrapping for other foods. In Japan, it is traditionally used to wrap sushi and rice balls, but if you want to be creative you can wrap any suitable food in it—a simple omelette, perhaps (see box, right). Another good way to use nori is as a garnish or flavouring. Pass the sheets carefully over a flame (or put them in a hot oven for a few minutes) until they become crisp, then crumble them onto salads or into soups.

Kombu (or konbu), also known as giant sea kelp, is also used for wrapping foods and is an essential component of Japanese stocks (dashi), which are made by soaking and heating strips of dried kombu in water. The kombu contains glutamic acid, which helps to soften other foods such as beans or chickpeas when they are cooked in the stock and is a valuable brain food in itself. Kombu is also rich in iodine and other minerals and is said to help reduce high blood

pressure. In the West, it is most commonly sold as dried strips or in powder form.

Other important Japanese seaweeds include wakame and hijiki. Wakame, the preferred seaweed for Japanese miso soup, is rich in calcium and vitamins B and C. Like kombu it can also act as a softener, and has a rather milder flavour. Hijiki contains a hundred times more calcium, weight for weight, than milk. It enjoys an excellent reputation in Japan for the improvement of skin and hair, and it has a gentle calming effect.

Soak dried wakame in water and it will expand to around ten times its size. It is rich in several key vitamins and minerals.

NORI-WRAPPED OMELETTE

Nori makes an ideal edible wrapper for foods because it sticks firmly to them, so it is easy to scoop portions of omelette on to a square of nori and fold it over to form a tasty parcel. Use a simple plain omelette, or fill it with ingredients such as peppers or pieces of cooked seafood. The inherent saltiness of the nori perfectly complements the omelette, and the parcel is a true brain food, with vitamins and minerals from the nori and protein and lecithin from the eggs.

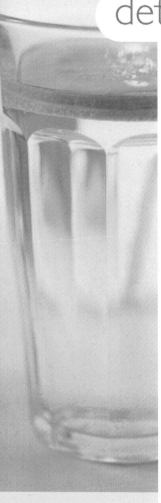

detoxing

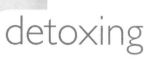

Cleansing your digestive system—whether or not you've been indulging in a diet high in sugars and fats or just want to give yourself an internal clear out—will definitely make you feel happier. The liver is a highly efficient detoxifying organ; it is very tough and able to repair itself from injuries. However, its strength is not inexhaustible and a continued assault on it, especially with well-known toxins such as alcohol in high levels, can take its toll. The kidneys, too, are important for flushing out toxins in the urine, and finally a properly functioning intestine is essential. It has long been recognized that the proper functioning of these organs has an important effect on the mental faculties, not simply when the organs begin to fail and toxins accumulate in the brain, but in everyday temper and mood. The mechanisms that control the production and transmission of neurotransmitters are finely balanced and they easily can be undermined by an overload of toxic material.

Toxic substances

Too much of anything can prove toxic to a sluggish digestive system and this is particularly true of caffeinated and alcoholic drinks and foods that are highly refined, high in animal or processed fats or sugar, and low in fibre.

Even if you have a normally functioning digestive system, periods of stress can make it less effective, and if the liver becomes overloaded you will be left with an excess of oxidants—harmful molecules that damage cell membranes. These can interefere with the transmission of messages in the brain.

In addition to ingesting toxins in the food we eat, we're also exposed to many external toxins, such as chemicals in car exhaust, that find their way into our systems. Well-known toxic substances include lead, mercury, copper, cadium and aluminium—some or all of which can be found in amalgam fillings, cooking pots, cigarette smoke, car exhaust and contaminated fish. Toxic metals have been implicated in a number of problems involving low mood, fatigue and poor mental function.

Doing a detox

Some authorities recommend a comprehensive detoxification about twice a year—in spring and autumn. The detoxification regime can last about two weeks and involves fasting, or almost fasting, coupled with the use of special teas. Such a regime is commonly known as a spagyric tea detoxification.

However, not everyone is either willing or able to follow such a regime, and we believe that it is possible to exert an important positive effect on one's

WATER

Essential to the optimal functioning of your digestive system, this is the ideal detox drink. A lack of water in the diet will result in the production of dry, compacted stools that can be painful to pass. It is recommended that you drink about four pints of water daily and more if you eat a lot of salty food or regularly drink large amounts of caffeine-rich or carbonated beverages. Some mineral waters are particularly low in minerals and many people argue—on not very much hard evidence—that one should drink waters that are slightly alkaline (pH >7), rather than slightly acid.

mental and physical wellbeing using a simpler regime over a much shorter time. This regime is primarily for otherwise healthy people who perhaps feel run down or over-stressed, for example, to cleanse their systems as part of a regular pick-me-up. The basic idea is to cut out caffeine (tea, coffee, colas), alcohol, smoking, and all "recreational" drugs. Proteins, dairy products and most grains should be reduced to a minimum or cut out altogether. Processed and fried foods and nuts should also be avoided. The conditions should be similar to fasting or almost fasting. The underlying principle is that what you eat and drink during the detoxification should involve nutrients that protect the liver and kidneys and antioxidants that can stimulate the body's own detoxification efforts.

Good food choices

We suggest that teas and fruit and vegetable juices form the basis of your detoxification plan. Green tea is full of antioxidants, and organic lemon, orange and lime juices also are good choices. Grapefruit juice, however, may interact with some prescription drugs in the liver.

Vegetables rich in antioxidants include carrots, celery, beetroot, tomatoes, spinach, lettuce and watercress, along with parsley, turmeric and cumin. Vitamin C, either in the form of citrus juice or vitamin supplements, as well as Vitamin E, can be important additions.

During the detoxification you should drink plenty of water. Some vegetables, such as asparagus and artichoke, as well as herbal teas, especially dandelion tea, are mildly diuretic and increase the flow of urine. This is where they can score most clearly in detoxification.

We recommend this detoxification period to last for at least twenty-four

HELPFUL HERBS

The best detoxification teas contain antioxidant-rich herbs such as dandelion root, ginger, spearmint, peppermint, burdock root, liquorice and sage. Proprietary herbal teas containing these components are readily available in health food shops, pharmacies and supermarkets.

Two other herbs seem to be particularly efficient at protecting the liver. These are milk thistle (*Silybum marianum*: with the active liver-protecting ingredient silymarin) and mugwort (*Artemesia vulgaris*).

Aloe vera tablets and liquorice root (*Glycyrrhiza glabra*) are also helpful, but bear in mind that these compounds can interfere with other prescribed medications and should not be used for long periods. In particular, milk thistle can interact with common (typical, first generation) antipsychotic drugs, and probably other antipsychotics as well.

hours, but probably not longer than 2–3 days. It is important that the cure is not more stressful to the body than the condition that it is designed to treat.

As long as you drink plenty of water, you should not come to any harm even if you prolong this period. The key, as in everything, is moderation.

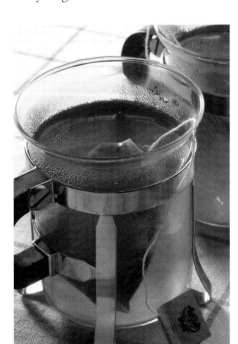

Green tea is rich in antioxidants, which are part of the body's natural defence mechanism and help to neutralise free radicals.

quick and easy ways of improving your favourite foods

To get more from the dishes you eat on a regular basis, there are two basic approaches, substitution and augmentation. "Substitution" means simply that you replace one or more of your usual ingredients with a healthier or superior item; "augmentation" means that you add an additional ingredient.

For example, you may find that foods rich in the amino acid tryptophan improve your sleep (see page 13). Tryptophan is the basic constituent of the neurotransmitter serotonin, which is of central importance in both mood and the sleep-wake cycle. So if you usually eat fruit with your evening meal, it makes sense to include bananas, which are rich in tryptophan. Bananas are also rich in carbohydrates, which help to increase the amount of tryptophan that is absorbed by the gut.

One problem you should be aware of is that processed foods have lost many of their vitamins, especially B vitamins. Vitamins B_1, B_6 and biotin are important in maintaining the function of neurotransmitters, as well as the energy-producing ability of the cells of the body. If you often eat rice dishes, for example, it's important to use brown rice, instead of white. Brown rice retains both the bran and germ of the rice kernel and is rich in nutrients; white rice is just starch.

It shouldn't be a problem to liven up salad dressings, for example, with a sprinkling of sunflower seeds, or to strew some chopped almonds over most green vegetables. Both of these are high in tryptophan. Or, bump up your magnesium intake by adding grated courgettes to pancakes, omelettes, or teabreads and meatloaves.

foods to substitute

- Turkey for chicken (more serotonin, selenium and B vitamins)
- Venison for beef (less fat, more B vitamins)
- Yoghurt for sour cream (more vitamins, less "bad" fat)
- Kale for lettuce (more serotonin and minerals, slower release of sugar)

- Green tea for black tea (contains antioxidants and helps the body to retain vitamin C)
- Bulgur for white rice (high in potassium and B vitamins)
- Sweet potatoes for potatoes (high concentration of vitamin A and potassium)

- Bok choy for white/green cabbage (high in betacarotene, vitamin C, potassium and calcium)
- Salmon for sea bass (richer in omega 3 fatty acids, iodine)
- Pacific salmon for Atlantic salmon (more retinol for vitamin A production)

- Low- or no-sodium salt for salt (may reduce high blood pressure)
- Sea salt (iodized) for table salt (boosts thyroid gland)
- Whole-grain bread for ordinary bread (slower energy release)
- Berries for grapes (slower energy release)

foods to add

FOR EXTRA FOLATE
Sunflower seeds
Peanuts
Wheat germ
Walnuts
Almonds
Mushrooms

FOR EXTRA TRYPTOPHAN
Peanuts
Eggs
Sunflower seeds

FOR EXTRA OMEGA 3
Fatty acids
Sunflower oil
Purslane
Tuna

FOR EXTRA SELENIUM
Onions
Wheat germ
Brazil nuts
Bran
Orange juice

FOR EXTRA CHROMIUM
Brewer's yeast
Wheat bran
Wheat germ
Green pepper
Cornmeal

FOR EXTRA VITAMIN B$_6$
Sunflower seeds
Toasted wheat germ
Walnuts
Raisins

Essential Seed Mix

Add this to your salads, breakfast cereals and cooked vegetables, and to sauces to ensure you get all the essential micro-minerals on a daily basis.

> Linseed (flaxseeds)
> Sesame seeds
> Sunflower seeds
> Pumpkin seeds

Combine equal amounts of the above four seeds and, in a blender or grinder, work until finely mixed. Store in a lidded container in a dark place and use within six weeks.

Miso Mix

A couple of spoonfuls in soups, stews, stocks, sauces, dressings, dips and spreads will ensure you get all the B vitamins you need. Don't add any extra salt.

> 3 tablespoons watercress
> 1 teaspoon ground cumin
> 125ml/4fl oz sesame oil
> 140g/5oz organic barley miso

Chop the watercress finely and mix with the ground cumin. Place in a lidded jar or bottle and add the sesame oil and barley miso. Shake to combine. Store in the refrigerator for up to two weeks and use as needed.

Miso is a textured vegetable protein made from fermented soya beans. Miso soup is central to the Japanese diet, and has been linked to lower rates of breast cancer.

Crumble Mix

Sugar-free and absolutely delicious, this can be poured over any type of fruit and baked until it's crunchy.

> 100g/3½oz plain sugar-free biscuits
> Juice of 2 medium-sized
>   organic oranges
> 3 tablespoons sugar-free peach jam
> 85ml/3fl oz maple syrup
> 55g/2oz flaked almonds

Wrap the biscuits in a large cotton tea towel, and then crush them to fine crumbs with a rolling pin. In a small mixing bowl, stir together the orange juice, jam and maple syrup. Pour it over your choice of fruit—for example, 450g (1lb) each organic apples and pears, coarsely chopped. Then sprinkle over the biscuit crumbs and flaked almonds. Bake in the oven at 180°C for 20–25 minutes.

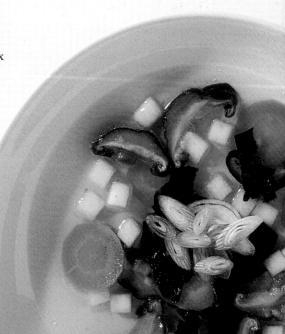

cooking as therapy

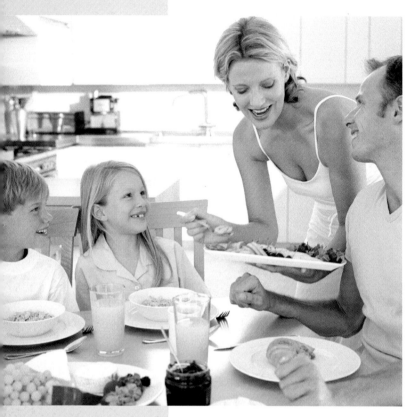

The main approach in this book is, of course, to look at the mental health effects of different nutrients and food supplements and to ensure that our choice of recipes provides readers not only with food that is delicious but mood improving as well. But cooking food has mental health benefits, too. The potential therapeutic effect of cooking, if we take cooking to incorporate the selection of the food, its preparation and, of course, the eating, is immense.

In modern life, it is all too easy for meal times to become rushed, unsocial affairs. Individuals who live on their own, particularly if they work during the day, may exist entirely on quick lunch breaks of ready-prepared food and dinners of microwave meals. But families, too, tend to eat separately today. In spite of wide recognition of the importance of a family meal time, all too often, a parent or parents will sit down to a solitary TV dinner while any offspring do the same in their own rooms. Such a situation is wide-ranging in its negative effects on individuals, the family, and society as a whole.

The beneficial effects

In order to cook, you need to be able to follow a recipe. The recipes in this book have been carefully tested and written with the average cook in mind; none of them should present any difficulty. However, concentrating on a meal and its preparation is a very useful way of disconnecting from any troubles bothering you, and allows you to direct your attention to the immediate task in hand. It's not that this kind of cooking requires profound intellectual skills, rather that cooking is a craft with a well-known series of techniques that anyone can learn, and creating a dish is in itself therapeutic. It is much easier to learn by doing rather than simply by reading. Learning anything helps to maintain cognitive function and contributes to mental fitness.

Eating yourself happy, by following the recipes in this book, is a practical way of learning not only about nutrition and the importance of different nutrients and supplements, but also how your brain works. You also should benefit from the knowledge that what you are making is going to be better for you and those that you love. If we are what we eat, then eating the recipes in this book is going to make you a much happier person.

Enhancing your skills

We are firmly of the view that the best ingredients are fresh, seasonal and additive-free. To put this into practice, you need to learn about the seasonal changes in food, how to assess the freshness of food products and how to read food labels. Without realizing it, you are also learning a great deal about the natural world in all its diversity.

Cooking requires basic skills of manual dexterity, and the hand-eye coordination involved helps to keep the mind agile. Other skills required include time management and attention to detail, and cooking makes a fuller use of your senses than you would obtain from reheating and eating a ready-made meal. Cooking also has myriad benefits for mood. Even if you live alone, cooking can be a pleasurable activity. Look on eating alone not as a chore but as a gift to yourself, as you might consider a cocktail or a warm bath at the end of the day. And, if you are lucky enough to be cooking for other people, then this act of making others happy will make you happy, too.

Food and wellbeing

Preparing food for others, especially loved ones, is more than simply putting plates on the table, or preparing a meal of aphrodisiac food. Care in planning a meal, its setting, the gathering of ingredients, their preparation and service is a loving act that makes the giver feel good, too. Eating together cements relationships and is conducive to good mental health and wellbeing.

The converse is also true. If your gift of food is ignored or undervalued, it is as if part of you is being ignored or undervalued in a way different from ordinary ingratitude. In other words, food is a basis of reciprocity, or give and take, in a relationship.

Cooking also can be an important social activity. Even if you live alone, if you become interested in cooking you can develop interpersonal skills and increase your self-confidence. Cooking with others can allow you to expand social networks by attending cooking classes, or by cooking for communal meals.

COLOUR HEALING

While the food that you eat is very important, so too is the setting in which you eat it. The use of colour is widely recognized to have a positive effect on mood, with varying shades having a surprising influence on the atmosphere and ambience in which you eat. If you want a casual and relaxed family gathering, try pale yellows and creams in your colour scheme for a tension-free meal. If you have passion in mind, choose vivid, hot colours such as purples or reds to increase the erotic ambience. Silver, gold, light grey or off-white are perfect for a more formal occasion, but add a splash of strong colour such as maroon to make your table really sparkle.

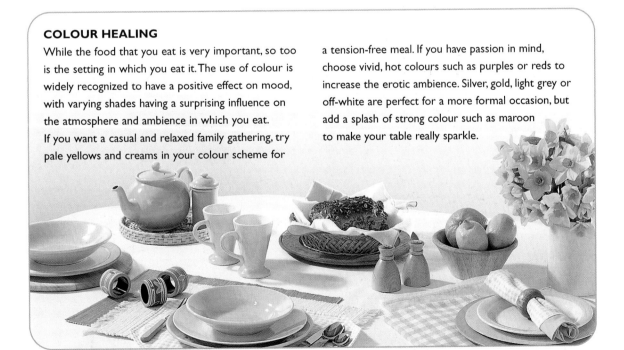

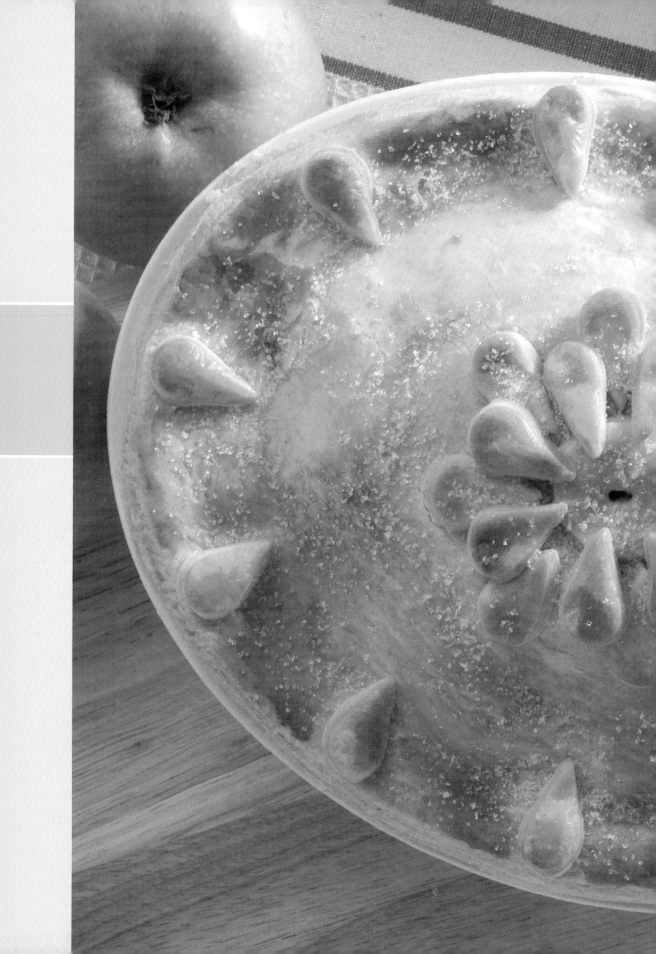

6

MOOD-ENHANCING RECIPES

We hope that you enjoy trying these recipes, which have been designed to complement the advice found in the previous chapters. Most of the ingredients are readily available, but if you find some difficult to source in supermarkets, make use of your local health food shop, which should be able to point you in the right direction, and also use the internet, a valuable tool for sourcing foodstuffs and supplements.

breakfast

Skipping breakfast is a feature of modern life, but you lose out in terms of poor concentration etc., over the morning. Choosing foods with a low to medium glycaemic index allows more even glucose levels to boost concentration.

scrambled eggs with portobello mushrooms

This dish is rich in brain food. Eggs are a good source of protein, and contain lecithin for memory, and eggs and mushrooms contain useful quantities of mood-boosting tryptophan, selenium and folate, as well as antioxidants.

SERVES 2
COOKING TIME 10 MINUTES

15g/½oz butter
2 free-range eggs, beaten
4 tablespoons olive oil
2 garlic cloves, sliced
200g/7oz portobello mushrooms, sliced
1 tablespoon parsley, chopped
Sea salt and black pepper

1 Heat the butter in a heavy-based saucepan. When it has melted, add the beaten eggs, stirring continuously to prevent them sticking. When the egg is cooked through but creamy, set aside.
2 Using another heavy-based saucepan heat the olive oil and add the garlic slices. Fry over a medium heat for 5 minutes until softened. Add the sliced mushrooms and cook for a further 5 minutes.
3 Stir in the eggs and chopped parsley until combined, add salt and black pepper to taste, and serve.

creamy scrambled eggs with smoked trout

Another recipe utilizing the brain-boosting potential of eggs. The trout is rich in omega-3 fatty acids. As well as protecting the body's cells by mopping up free radicals, rosemary contains phytochemicals—natural antibiotics—and is a valuable folk remedy for headache.

SERVES 4
COOKING TIME 15 MINUTES

100g/3½oz smoked trout fillet
8 free-range eggs
100g/3½oz firm cream cheese, cut into small pieces
½ red onion, finely chopped
A handful of fresh rosemary, chopped (or 1 level teaspoon, dried)
1 teaspoon olive oil

1 Break the trout into small pieces. Whisk the eggs in a large bowl until well blended. Stir in the trout, cream cheese, red onion and rosemary.
2 Heat the oil in a large non-stick frying pan over a medium heat.
3 Pour in the egg mixture and turn down the heat to low. Cook, stirring continuously, for 5 minutes until the mixture is lightly scrambled. Remove the pan from the heat and serve at once.

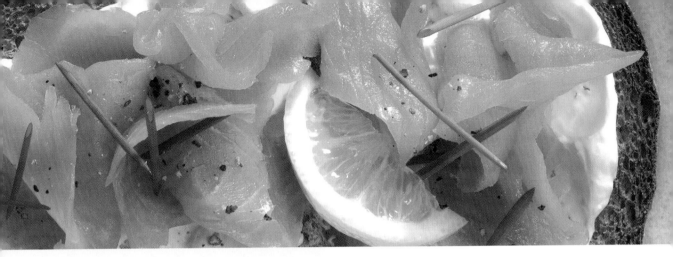

toast with cream cheese and smoked salmon

This simple but delicious breakfast is full of calcium, proteins, vitamins and omega-3 fatty acids that will boost brain function. Salmon—ideally not farmed, unless to organic standards—is a rich source of omega-3 fatty acids and tryptophan, as well as folate.

SERVES 2
COOKING TIME 5 MINUTES

2 slices wholemeal bread
2 tablespoons cream cheese
2 slices of wild smoked salmon
Lemon juice (optional)
Sea salt and black pepper
Chopped chives, to garnish

1   Toast the bread, spread the cream cheese on the toast and top with a slice of smoked salmon.
2   Add a squeeze of lemon juice (if using) and salt and pepper to taste. Garnish with chives and serve.

muesli

This muesli is packed with goodness and is a great all-round brain food. The cereal flakes are low to medium on the glycaemic index, so that your glucose levels rise steadily to keep you going over the hardest morning.

MAKES ABOUT 40 SERVINGS
COOKING TIME 10 MINUTES

225g/8oz rolled oat flakes
175g/6oz rolled wheat flakes
175g/6oz rolled rye flakes
175g/6oz rolled barley flakes
100g/3½oz sunflower seeds
100g/3½oz flaxseeds (linseeds)
100g/3½oz almonds, chopped
100g/3½oz hazelnuts, chopped
100g/3½oz dried dates, chopped
100g/3½oz dried apricots, chopped
100g/3½oz stoned, dried, ready-to-eat prunes, chopped
100g/3½oz raisins

1   Mix all the ingredients together and store in an airtight container. Serve with fresh fruit and low-fat natural yoghurt, low-fat milk or fruit juice.

power brunch

This traditional breakfast is popular, but has had a bad press. However, it contains highly nutritious foods, and can help boost the mood through tryptophan, selenium and folate. Portobello mushrooms are rich in vitamins, especially vitamin D and niacin. This is valuable not only in reducing "bad" cholesterol (LDL) but also, unlike most foods, increasing levels of "good" cholesterol (HDL).

SERVES 2
COOKING TIME 15 MINUTES

2 garlic sausages
2 slices of rindless bacon
2 vine tomatoes, halved
2 Portobello mushrooms
Olive oil for brushing
1 teaspoon vinegar
2 free-range eggs
1 small can of baked beans

1   Heat the grill to a medium heat and place the sausages, bacon, tomatoes and mushrooms on the grill rack. Brush the mushrooms lightly with olive oil and grill everything for 4–5 minutes on each side.
2   Meanwhile, heat a shallow pan of water to simmering point and add the vinegar. Break each egg into a cup and gently slide them, one at a time, into the water. Keeping the water at a steady temperature, spoon a little water over the yolks until they are cooked through.
3   Heat the beans and serve with toast.

spinach tortilla

SERVES 3
COOKING TIME 25 MINUTES

100g/3½oz spinach
3 tablespoon olive oil
½ onion, chopped
1 glove garlic, chopped
3 eggs, beaten
Grated cheese for topping (optional)
1 handful fresh parsley, chopped (or 1 teaspoon dried parsley)

1   Steam the spinach for 3–4 minutes.
2   Meanwhile, heat the oil in a large frying pan and fry the onion and garlic until translucent.
3   Chop the spinach and add to the frying pan. Cook for 2 minutes.
4   Add the beaten eggs and continue cooking. When the mixture is almost set, grate the cheese over the top (optional). Fold mixture in half, and fry for about 3 minutes, until golden brown. Turn onto a warm plate, sprinkle the parsley over the top and eat immediately.

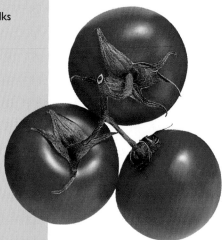

broccoli smoothie

This is one of the most energizing breakfasts-in-a-glass, packed with mood boosting minerals, and with a low GI.

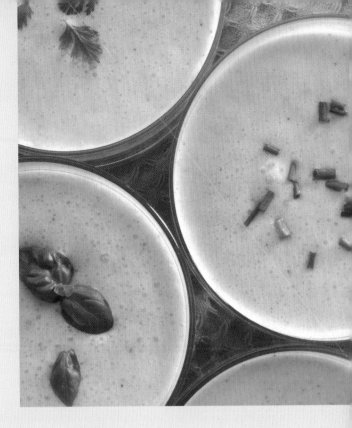

SERVES 2-4
COOKING TIME 5 MINUTES

150g/5½oz steamed broccoli
150g/5½oz tofu (reserve the liquid in the pack and make up to ½ litre with cold semi-skimmed milk)
Salt and freshly ground black pepper, to taste
selection of finely chopped herbs (parsley, coriander, oregano, chives), to taste

1 Place all the ingredients in a blender or food processor and whiz together until smooth.
2 Add seasoning and herbs, to taste. Serve immediately.

banana smoothie

Bananas are good sources of magnesium, potassium, vitamin B$_6$, folate and antioxidants. Although a good source of carbohydrate, banana has a low to medium glycaemic index, providing sustained energy. Peanut butter is rich in protein, magnesium and vital trace elements such as manganese and zinc.

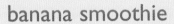

SERVES 4
COOKING TIME 5 MINUTES

2 bananas, chopped
2 tablespoons peanut butter
55g/2oz silken tofu lite
2 tablespoons chocolate syrup or 1 tbsp of cocoa
1.2 litres/2 pints skimmed milk

1 Place all the ingredients in a blender or food processor and whiz together until smooth.
2 Pour into four glasses and chill for at least 1 hour, then serve.

soy smoothie

This is a refreshing, magnesium-, folate- and antioxidant-rich drink, an ideal mood-enhancing combination. This smoothie is also good for physical health and can reduce cholesterol in the blood and improve the digestion. The probiotic yoghurt (see page 92) is a good source of vitamins B and K, important after a course of antibiotic medication.

SERVES 4
COOKING TIME 5 MINUTES

175ml/6fl oz silken tofu lite
2 tablespoons fat-free, probiotic yoghurt
115g/4oz fresh or frozen strawberries or raspberries, hulled

1 Place all the ingredients in a blender or food processor and whiz together until smooth.
2 Pour into four glasses and serve immediately.

light snacks and soups

It's good to have some nutritious but quick and easy-to-prepare snack recipes to fall back on when you need them most. For many, soup is the ultimate comforter, so make your own and reap the rewards.

pan tomate with anchovies and tapenade

This simple dish is a favourite on the east coast of Spain. Anchovies are especially rich in omega-3 fatty acids, magnesium, selenium, tryptophan, folate, and iodine, all of which boost mood and concentration. Wheat-germ oil contains especially high levels of vitamin E, a potent source of antioxidants.

SERVES 2
COOKING TIME 5 MINUTES

2 slices wholemeal bread
1 garlic clove, cut in half
1 tomato, halved
1 teaspoon olive oil or wheat-germ oil
4 anchovies in vinegar
2 tablespoons tapenade
Black pepper to taste

1 Rub the slices of bread all over with the garlic clove. Rub the tomato halves into each slice of bread. Then drizzle the bread with the oil.
2 Add 2 anchovies to each slice of bread, then cover with 1 tablespoon of tapenade. Sprinkle with black pepper and serve.

endive with anchovies, cheese and white wine

Endive is rich in folate, vitamin C and trace elements that enhance mood, and also contains prebiotics (see page 93).

SERVES 4
COOKING TIME 10 MINUTES

For the filling:
125g/4½oz Stilton or strong, blue-veined cheese
125ml/4fl oz white wine
1 head endive, separated into single leaves
4 anchovy fillets in oil, sliced in half
8 walnuts, halved

For the vinaigrette:
3 tablespoons olive oil
1 tablespoon sherry vinegar
1 tablespoon cold water
1 garlic clove, crushed
1 teaspoon Dijon mustard

1 Place the cheese and white wine into a food processor and whiz until smooth.
2 Put a tablespoon of the cheese mixture into each endive leaf and top with an anchovy fillet and two half walnuts.
3 Put all the ingredients for the vinaigrette into a screw-top jar and shake well to mix. Trickle over the endive and serve.

salad with asparagus, tuna and anchovies

Full of vital trace elements, this dish improves mood and reduces levels of anxiety. New potatoes have a medium glycaemic index, and contain small amounts of lithium, a drug used, in much higher doses, to help mood disorders.

SERVES 4
COOKING TIME 30 MINUTES

For the dressing:
2 tablespoons olive oil
Salt, to taste
1 tablespoon balsamic vinegar

For the salad:
500g/1lb 2oz new potatoes, scrubbed
450g/1lb fresh young asparagus, washed
4 free-range eggs
1 Romaine lettuce, washed and torn
4 vine tomatoes, quartered
3 spring onions, chopped
200g/7oz can olives stuffed with anchovies
200g/7oz can tuna in water or brine
55g/2oz can anchovies
Black pepper, to taste

1 To make the dressing, whisk together the olive oil, salt and balsamic vinegar until well combined.
2 To make the salad, put the potatoes in a large saucepan, cover with cold water and bring to the boil. Reduce the heat and cook for about 15 minutes or until tender. Drain well, slice and leave to cool.
3 Steam the asparagus until tender. Boil the eggs for 10 minutes. Remove from the heat, peel, chop and leave to cool.
4 Place the sliced potatoes, eggs, lettuce, tomatoes, spring onions and olives in a serving dish, and pour the dressing over the salad mixture.
5 Decorate the salad with the asparagus, tuna fish and anchovies. Season with black pepper and serve.

red pepper humous

Humous is derived from chickpeas, a rich source of plant protein and phytoestrogens that can boost mood.

SERVES 2
COOKING TIME 25 MINUTES

1 red pepper, sliced in half
4 tablespoons of humous
Granary or wholemeal toast to serve

1 Place the pepper halves under a hot grill for about 10 minutes or until the skin is black. Cover with a clean wet cloth or place in a plastic bag and allow to cool for about 10 minutes.
2 Remove the skin from the pepper and roughly chop the flesh. Stir into the humous and serve with wholemeal toast.

pisto

SERVES 4
COOKING TIME 30 MINUTES

5 tablespoons olive oil
2 medium onions, chopped
1 clove garlic, finely chopped
1 red pepper, cubed
1 green pepper, cubed
2 small courgettes, cubed
1 400g/14oz can chopped tomatoes
Salt and freshly ground black pepper to taste
1 400g/14oz can artichoke hearts, drained and cubed

1 Heat the oil in a large frying pan and fry the onions and garlic until translucent.
2 Add the peppers, courgettes and tomatoes, season to taste, and cook through on a medium heat for about 15 minutes, until the vegetables are soft.
3 Add the cubed artichoke hearts and cook for a further 5 minutes. Serve immediately.

spanish omelette

This recipe contains a great deal of brain food, including choline and lecithin from the eggs and vitamins and trace elements from the potatoes and vegetables. The glycaemic index is low to medium.

SERVES 4
COOKING TIME 30 MINUTES

8 tablespoons olive oil
350g/12oz floury potatoes, peeled and chopped into small cubes
2 small red onions, peeled and finely chopped
6 medium free-range eggs
Salt and freshly ground black pepper to taste
115g/4oz fresh (or frozen) peas, cooked
115g/4oz broccoli florets, cooked
Mixed green salad, to serve

1   Heat half the oil in a non-stick frying pan over a medium heat. Add the potatoes and onions and cook for 10–15 minutes. Set the potatoes and onions aside and discard any remaining oil.
2   Beat the eggs with the seasoning, then stir in the onions, potatoes, peas and broccoli.
3   Heat the remaining oil in a clean pan, add the mixture and cook over a medium heat for 12–15 minutes until the top of the omelette begins to set and the bottom is cooked. Place the pan under a hot grill and cook for about 10 minutes until the top of the omelette is set.
4   Cut into wedges and serve with a mixed salad.

turkey stir-fry

SERVES 4
COOKING TIME 30 MINUTES

450g/1lb skinless, boneless turkey breast, cut into strips
2 tablespoons olive oil
1 large onion, finely sliced
1 red pepper, finely sliced
1 yellow or orange pepper, finely sliced
1 large head of broccoli, cut into small florets
1 courgette, sliced
2 cloves garlic, crushed
1 tablespoon sherry
1 teaspoon sesame oil
2 tablespoons soy sauce
4 spring onions, cut into chunky pieces
55g/2oz flaked almonds

1   Place a non-stick wok or large non-stick frying pan over a high heat and dry fry the turkey in batches until browned. Set aside.
2   Heat the olive oil in the same pan over a medium heat and stir-fry the onion and peppers for 5 minutes. Add the broccoli and stir-fry for a further 5 minutes. Add the courgette and garlic and stir-fry for three minutes more.
3   Return the turkey to the pan and stir-fry over a medium heat for 5 minutes. Stir in the sherry, sesame oil and soy sauce and cook for a further 5 minutes, until the turkey is cooked through.
4   Stir in the spring onions. Transfer to individual dishes and scatter with the almonds to serve.

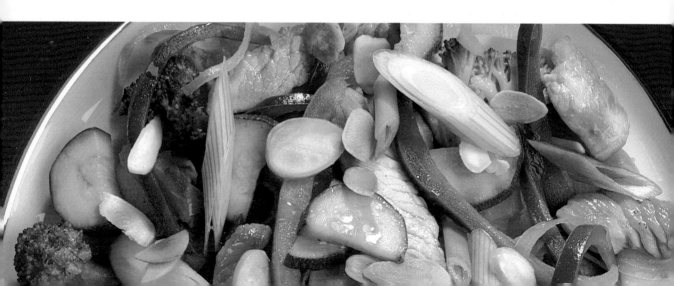

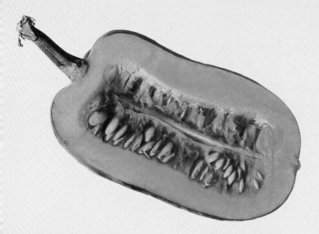

squash soup with saffron

Squashes are rich in fighter chemicals, including the important phytosterols. They have lots of calcium, iron, magnesium, manganese, phosphorus, selenium and zinc, as well as being packed with vitamins A, C and E.

SERVES 4
COOKING TIME 45 MINUTES

1 tablespoon olive oil
1 large onion, finely chopped
Large wedge of squash, (about 900g/2lbs) peeled, seeded and cubed
350g/12oz potatoes, peeled and cubed
1 clove garlic, crushed
1 teaspoon saffron strands
Small bunch parsley, chopped
1 litre/1¾ pints vegetable stock
Salt and freshly ground black pepper
Grated cheddar cheese

1   Heat the oil in a large saucepan and add the onion. Cook for about 5 minutes until soft. Add the squash, potatoes, garlic, saffron strands and parsley and cook, stirring, for 10–15 minutes until the squash begins to soften.
2   Pour in the stock and add salt and pepper. Bring to a boil, then simmer for 20–25 minutes.
3   Transfer to a blender and purée until smooth. Reheat, but do not boil, and serve topped with a sprinkling of cheese.

gazpacho

A classic summer soup, full of antioxidants—an ideal detoxing drink.

SERVES 4
COOKING TIME 15 MINUTES

1kg/2lb 4oz ripe tomatoes, peeled and chopped
1 small cucumber, peeled and chopped
1 small green pepper, chopped
2 cloves garlic, crushed
Salt and pepper
4 tablespoons balsamic vinegar
125ml/4fl oz olive oil
Chopped cucumber, onion, red or green pepper, tomatoes and hard-boiled eggs, to serve

1   Place the chopped tomatoes, cucumber, green pepper, crushed garlic, salt and pepper and balsamic vinegar in a blender and blend thoroughly.
2   Gradually add the olive oil and continue to blend the mixture until smooth. If the consistency is too thick, dilute it with a little water.
3   Chill well before serving. When ready to serve, add chopped cucumber, onion, red or green pepper, hard-boiled eggs and tomatoes.

chicken soup

Very rich in tryptophan and low in fat, this soup is the ultimate comfort food.

SERVES 6
COOKING TIME 3 HOURS

250g/9oz chicken legs and thighs, with bones
1½ litres/2¾ pints water
1 stick celery, roughly chopped
1 medium onion, chopped
1 medium leek, sliced
2 medium carrots, sliced
2 cloves garlic, crushed
1 bay leaf

1 Put all the ingredients in a large saucepan, bring to a boil very slowly over a low heat, cover and simmer for about 3 hours, until the chicken is very tender and almost falling from the bones.
2 Over a large bowl, strain the soup through a colander. Remove and reserve the chicken pieces but discard the other solid ingredients.
3 Using a slotted spoon, skim any fat from the surface and return the soup to the washed saucepan.
4 Discard the chicken bones and remove any skin, then mince the chicken, return it to the soup and reheat. Serve with crusty bread.

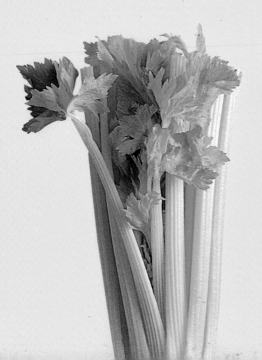

shrimp soup

Shrimps are full of vitamins and minerals, including iodine, copper and fluoride. They contain mood-enhancing selenium.

SERVES 6
COOKING TIME 50 MINUTES

85g/3oz butter
1 medium carrot, chopped
1 medium onion, finely chopped
1 stick celery, finely chopped
675g/1½lb raw or cooked shrimps
700ml/1¼ pint fish stock
1 bay leaf
200ml/7fl oz dry white wine
100ml/3½fl oz dry sherry
25g/1oz plain flour
300ml/10fl oz semi-skimmed milk
150ml/5fl oz double cream
Salt and freshly ground black pepper

1 Melt 25g/1oz of the butter in a medium-sized saucepan. Add the carrot, onion and celery and cook over a medium heat for 3–4 minutes.
2 If you are using raw shrimps, add them to the pan and turn them over in the butter for 5 minutes, until they are pink, before adding the fish stock, bay leaf wine and sherry (if you are using cooked shrimps, add them at the same time as the stock etc.). Bring to the boil and simmer for 20 minutes.
3 Transfer the soup to a blender and liquidize for a few seconds until coarsely blended, not completely smooth. Pour the mixture into a sieve and press all the liquid through the sieve with the back of a ladle.
4 Melt the remaining butter in another saucepan, stir in the flour and cook for 30 seconds. Gradually add the milk and then the strained soup and simmer over a low heat for 20 minutes, stirring occasionally. Whisk in the cream and season with salt and pepper. Serve with a few peeled shrimps in the bottom of each bowl before adding the soup.

main dishes

As fish is such a valuable source of protein and omega-3 and 6 fatty acids, we've given a number of delicious fish recipes in this section. Many people are wary of cooking with fish, but don't be put off—it's easy and highly nutritious.

lemon sole with almonds

Another serotonin factory! Sole and almonds are rich in omega-3 and omega-9 fatty acids, magnesium, folate, trace elements and antioxidants. Spinach is especially rich in vitamins, including folate, and minerals.

SERVES 4
COOKING TIME 25 MINUTES

500ml/18fl oz fish stock
25g/1oz butter
4 lemon sole fillets, about 125g/4½oz each
1 tablespoon double cream
2 drops of almond essence
1 tablespoon lemon juice
pinch fresh thyme
1 bay leaf
White pepper
200g/7oz baby spinach, washed

1 Place the fish stock in a small saucepan and bring to the boil.
2 Heat the butter in a frying pan. Add the fish and cook with the skin down for two minutes or until brown. Add the fish stock, cream, almond essence, lemon juice, thyme and bay leaf, bring to the boil and cook for 5 minutes. Season with white pepper.
3 Place the spinach in a large saucepan and cook until just wilted. Spoon the spinach on to a serving dish, place the fish on top and spoon over the sauce.

calamari a la romana

Calamari (young squid) are a good source of choline and selenium. Soy oil is rich in omega-6 fatty acids and antioxidants (but olive oil is a healthy substitute).

SERVES 4
COOKING TIME 10 MINUTES

350g/12oz squid, cleaned and cut into rings
Sea salt
55g/2oz seasoned flour
Soy oil for frying
1 lemon cut into wedges
Herb salad, to serve

1 Season the squid with a little salt and then toss in the seasoned flour until covered.
2 Put the soy oil in a large pan and heat to 190°C. Add the squid and fry for 1 minute, until crisp and golden.
3 Using a slotted spoon, remove the squid from the oil and drain on kitchen paper. Serve with lemon wedges and a herb salad.

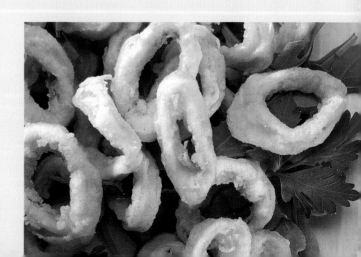

fisherman's pie

Another comforting favourite! The carbohydrates in the potatoes have a medium glycaemic index and also aid the absorption of tryptophan from the protein in the eggs and fish.

SERVES 4
COOKING TIME 1 HOUR 15 MINUTES

2 large free-range eggs
350g/12oz cod or haddock fillets
400ml/14fl oz semi-skimmed milk
1 bay leaf
5 black peppercorns
1 blade mace
25g/1oz butter
1 small leek, finely sliced
2 tablespoons plain flour
1 tablespoon capers, chopped
4 small gherkins, chopped
2 tablespoons chopped parsley
1 tablespoon lemon juice

For the topping:
900g/2lbs new potatoes, washed
85g/3oz low-fat soft cheese
4 tablespoons milk
Salt and freshly ground black pepper
55g/2oz Cheddar cheese, grated

1   Hard boil the eggs in a pan of simmering water for 10 minutes, drain and leave in cold water until cool.
2   Put the fish in a large saucepan. Add the milk, bay leaf, peppercorns and mace and bring to the boil. Cover and simmer gently for 10 minutes.
3   Set the fish aside to cool briefly and strain the cooking milk into a measuring jug, discarding the bay leaf, peppercorns and mace.
4   Cook the potatoes for 20–25 minutes or until tender. While the potatoes are cooking, shell the eggs, chop and set aside. Flake the fish into chunks, discarding any remaining bone and skin, and place in a large mixing bowl.
5   Heat the butter in a large saucepan and add the leek. Cook gently for 5 minutes, stirring, until tender. Stir in the flour and continue cooking for 2–3 minutes over a medium heat.
6   Gradually add the reserved milk, stirring into a smooth sauce. Bring to the boil, reduce the heat and simmer, stirring continuously, for 10–12 minutes. Remove the pan from the heat and set aside.
7   To make the topping, drain the cooked potatoes, and, with their skins still on, return them to the pan and mash thoroughly. Using a wooden spoon, beat in the soft cheese and milk. Season with salt and pepper and continue beating until light and fluffy.
8   Heat the oven to 200°C. Gently stir the eggs, fish, capers, gherkins, parsley and lemon juice into the sauce. Add salt and pepper to taste, then transfer to a large ovenproof dish. Top with the mashed potatoes and sprinkle with the grated cheese. Bake for 25 minutes until golden brown.

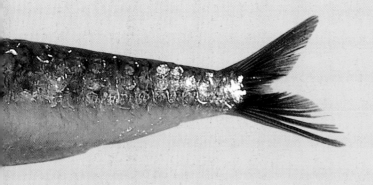

salmon in capers marinade and aubergine with miso

This delicious fusion dish is rich in omega-3 fatty acids, phytosterols and probiotics, as well as being packed with vitamins and minerals.

SERVES 2
COOKING TIME 30 MINUTES

2 salmon fillets, each weighing about 115g/4oz

For the marinade:
1 tablespoon lemon juice
1 tablespoon cider vinegar
1 tablespoon olive oil
1 tablespoon capers, chopped
1 tablespoon chopped parsley
Sea salt and freshly ground black pepper

For the aubergine mixture:
3 tablespoons olive oil
400g/14oz aubergine, peeled, cut in half lengthways and
  sliced into ½-inch thick pieces
4 tablespoons sake or white wine
150ml/5fl oz water
2 tablespoons miso paste

1   In a large bowl, mix together all the marinade ingredients. Pour over the salmon fillets, cover and marinate in the refrigerator for at least 30 minutes, overnight if possible.
2   Heat the olive oil in a large non-stick frying pan over a medium heat. Fry the aubergine for 3–4 minutes, add the sake or white wine and water and cook for a further 10 minutes. Add the miso paste and mix well.
3   When ready to cook the fish, heat the grill to medium hot. Remove the salmon fillets from the marinade and place them on a grill pan. Grill them for 7 minutes each side.
4   Spoon the aubergine mixture onto serving plates and top with the grilled fish.

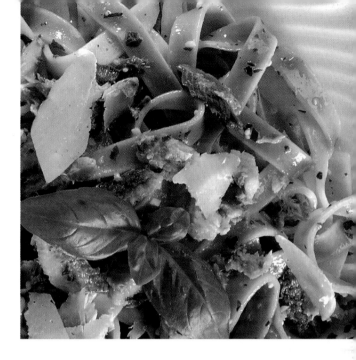

tagliatelle with sardines and pesto

Tagliatelle has a medium glycaemic index and is thus a good source of complex carbohydrates. Sardines are rich in omega-3 fatty acids and iron, and if you can eat the tiny bones they provide an excellent source of calcium.

SERVES 4
COOKING TIME 15 MINUTES

300g/10½oz dried tagliatelle
2 small cans sardines
2 tablespoons pesto sauce
1 tablespoon olive oil
1 clove garlic, finely minced
25g/1oz Parmesan cheese, grated

1   Bring a large pan of water to the boil, add the pasta and cook according to the packet instructions.
2   Put the sardines into a medium-sized bowl and mash with a fork. Add the pesto and combine well.
3   Drain the pasta, then return it to the pan and stir in the olive oil and the minced garlic. Then add the sardine mixture and combine well. Spoon into bowls, sprinkle with the grated Parmesan and serve.

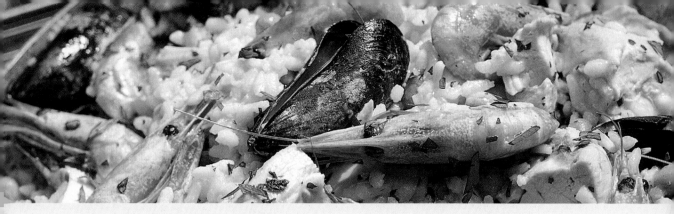

atlantic herrings with vine-ripened tomato sauce

Herrings provide one of the richest sources of omega-3 fatty acids, as well as antioxidants and iron. Thyme is rich in trace minerals and is a valuable digestive as well as having some effect in lowering blood cholesterol.

SERVES 4
COOKING TIME 30 MINUTES

For the sauce:
2 cloves garlic, crushed
2 tablespoons olive oil
2 tablespoons fresh parsley, chopped
1 tablespoon fresh thyme, chopped
2 tablespoons tomato purée
500g/1lb 2oz vine-ripened tomatoes, peeled, de-seeded and chopped

4 herrings, about 140g/5oz each, cleaned and trimmed
Salt and freshly ground black pepper, to taste
55g/2oz cheddar cheese, grated

1 To make the sauce, put all the ingredients in a food processor and blend until smooth. Place the mixture in a medium-sized pan. Cover the pan and cook over a medium heat for 10 minutes.
2 Pre-heat the grill to high and grill the herrings for 5 minutes on each side.
3 Place the herrings in an ovenproof dish and cover with the tomato sauce. Season to taste and sprinkle with cheese.
4 Place the dish under a hot grill for 10 minutes, until the cheese has melted. Serve.

manchego risotto with clams

Cheese is rich in calcium and trace elements. The addition of seaweed enriches the mood-elevating power of this dish (see page 98), and the clams provide selenium and omega-3 fatty acids.

SERVES 2
COOKING TIME 30 MINUTES

15g/½oz butter
1 small onion, finely chopped
115g/4oz risotto rice
600ml/1 pint hot vegetable stock
2 tablespoons grated Manchego cheese (if you can't find Manchego use Cheddar instead)
3 tablespoons clams, washed
2 tablespoons double cream
2 tablespoons fresh chives, chopped
White pepper and salt, to taste
Furikake or crumbled nori seaweed, to garnish

1 Heat the butter in large saucepan, add the onion and cook for 1–2 minutes. Add the rice and stir well to coat the grains. Cook for one minute.
2 Add the hot stock, a ladle at a time, and cook over a medium heat, stirring continuously until the stock becomes absorbed.
3 When the rice is just tender, remove from the heat and stir in the cheese, clams, cream and chives. Season to taste. Sprinkle over the Furikake or crumbled nori and serve.

paella

This is almost perfect brain food, as well as being comforting and delicious.

SERVES 4
COOKING TIME 45 MINUTES

5 tablespoons olive oil
1 medium onion, chopped
225g/8oz can tomatoes
1 medium red pepper
2 medium carrots, sliced
225g/8oz chicken, cut into small cubes
225g/8oz squid, cleaned and cut into rings
225g/8oz paella rice
450ml/16fl oz boiling water
1 heaped tablespoon bouillon powder
1kg/2lb 4oz fresh mussels (with shells), cleaned
500g/1lb 2oz fresh mussels (shelled)
1 clove garlic, sliced
Handful fresh parsley, chopped
1 teaspoon saffron strands
1 tablespoon melted butter
225g/8oz cooked prawns
225g/8oz fresh or frozen peas

1   Heat 1 tablespoon of the oil in a large, non-stick pan and fry the onions, tomatoes, pepper and carrot until the onion is translucent. Add the chicken cubes and squid rings and fry together for 5 minutes.
2   Add the rice and fry for 2 minutes, keeping the ingredients moving so that they do not stick.
3   Add the boiling water and bouillon powder and mix thoroughly. Add the remaining oil and allow the mixture to boil, then reduce the flame to medium and simmer for about 10 minutes.
4   Add the the mussels, garlic and parsley and simmer for a further 10 minutes.
5   Crush the saffron strands with one tablespoon of boiling water, then add the melted butter. Add this to the rice and mix carefully. Simmer for 5 minutes.
6   Add the prawns and peas and simmer for a further 5 minutes. Remove from the heat and let the paella rest for about 5 minutes before serving.

salpicón of chicken

This dish is loaded with vitamins, trace elements and antioxidants. Using turmeric instead of cumin in the dressing can aid digestion.

SERVES 4
COOKING TIME 30 MINUTES

2 carrots, sliced into thin strips
4 lettuce leaves, roughly chopped
4 Chinese cabbage leaves, sliced into bite-sized pieces
1 tomato, sliced
2 apples, diced
400g/14oz cooked chicken, sliced into thin strips

For the dressing:
Juice of 1 lemon
2 tablespoons olive oil
2 teaspoons Dijon mustard
5 tablespoons yoghurt
1 teaspoon cumin or turmeric
Salt

1   In a large pan of salted water cook the carrots for about 10 minutes, until just tender. Then drain and refresh them under cold water.
2   In a large bowl, mix the carrots, lettuce, cabbage, tomato and apples.
3   In a large bowl whisk together all the ingredients for the dressing, then add the chicken and mix well.
4   Place the salad mixture on serving plates, spoon the chicken mixture on top and serve.

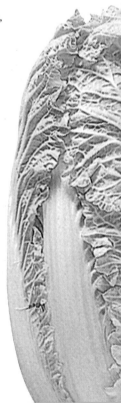

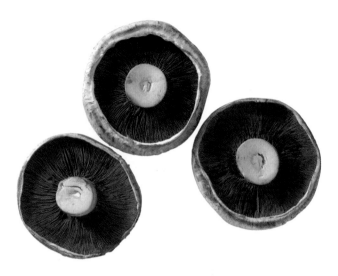

grilled beef with portobello mushrooms

Although too much beef is not a great idea, beef is rich in iron and folate—both very important in treating depression—and is full of vitamins, especially B_2 and B_3.

SERVES 2
COOKING TIME 10 MINUTES

For the marinade:
1 teaspoon fresh rosemary, chopped
2 fresh or 1 dried bay leaf
1 teaspoon onion, chopped
1 teaspoon fresh sage, chopped
1 teaspoon fresh basil, chopped
1 teaspoon Dijon mustard
1 teaspoon ground cumin
2 tablespoons olive oil

2 x organic steaks, cut from the topside, about 150g/5½oz each
2 cloves garlic, peeled and halved
Salt and freshly ground black pepper to taste
1 tablespoon olive oil

For the mushrooms:
200g/7oz Portobello mushrooms, stalks removed
1 clove garlic, peeled and crushed
Salt and freshly ground black pepper

1   Place all the ingredients for the marinade into a shallow dish and mix well. Using a small, sharp knife, score the steaks lightly on each side and rub them with the garlic. Sprinkle them with salt, pepper and oil on both sides. Place the steaks in the bowl with the marinade mixture, coating both sides, and chill in the fridge for at least 6 hours.
2   Wash and trim the mushrooms and sprinkle with the crushed garlic and salt and pepper. Heat the grill to medium/hot. Place the mushrooms and the steaks on the grill rack and grill for 5 minutes each side.
3   To serve, place the mushrooms rounded-side down on a warm plate and place the steak on top.

venison steaks

Venison is one of the healthiest red meats and one of the best for mood boosting—its high magnesium, selenium, folate and tryptophan content ensure that.

SERVES 2
COOKING TIME 10 MINUTES

2 venison steaks, about 150g/5½oz each
Olive oil for brushing

175g/6oz mixed salad leaves
200g/7oz can olives stuffed with anchovies
1 tablespoon olive oil
1 tablespoon balsamic vinegar
¼ teaspoon garlic purée
Salt and freshly ground black pepper, to taste

1   Heat the grill to hot. Brush the venison steaks lightly with olive oil and place them on the grill rack. Grill for 3 minutes on each side.
2   Put the salad leaves into a serving dish and add the olives. Whisk together the olive oil, balsamic vinegar, garlic purée and seasoning to taste. Drizzle over the salad. Serve with the venison steaks.

desserts

We've already looked at the beneficial effects of glucose and sugars, so what better way to enjoy the feel-good factor than with a delicious dessert? The recipes included here all have great mood-enhancing properties.

apple pie with cinnamon, hazelnuts and Cointreau

The apples help the amino acids from the breakdown of protein in the nuts to reach the brain, as well as providing a useful source of glucose and complex carbohydrates. The ingredients are rich in chromium, which helps in the absorption of tryptophan.

SERVES 4
COOKING TIME 50 MINUTES
(plus 1 hour chilling time)

675g/1lb 8oz cooking apples, peeled, cored and sliced
2 tablespoons caster sugar or sucralose (plus some
  for sprinkling)
¼ teaspoon ground cinnamon
2 tablespoons hazelnuts, chopped
1 tablespoon Cointreau (optional)
125g/4½oz plain flour
55g/2oz butter
Milk for brushing

1 Place the apple in a shallow bowl and add the sugar or sucralose, cinnamon, chopped hazelnuts and Cointreau, if using. Cover and set aside.
2 Put the flour and butter in a bowl. Rub the butter into the flour until the mixture resembles fine breadcrumbs. Gradually add cold water, about 3 tablespoons, until the mixture comes together. Wrap and chill for 30 minutes.

3 On a lightly floured surface, roll out the dough to about 6cm/2½in larger than the top of a 24 x 18cm/9½ x 7in pie dish. Cut a strip about 2.5cm/1in wide from around the edge of the pastry. Brush the rim of the pie dish with water and press the pastry strip onto it. Put the apple mixture into the pie dish, piling it high in the middle.
4 Dampen the pastry rim with water and cover with the pastry. Press the edge firmly to seal it well all round. Decorate the top with pastry shapes, make a hole in the middle for the steam to escape and chill for about 30 minutes. Heat the oven to 180°C.
5 Stand the pie on a baking tray to catch any juices. Brush the top with a little milk and bake for about 35 minutes until the top is pale golden and the fruit is bubbling inside.
6 Brush with a little milk and sprinkle with a little caster sugar then bake for a further 5 minutes. Serve with custard or fresh cream.

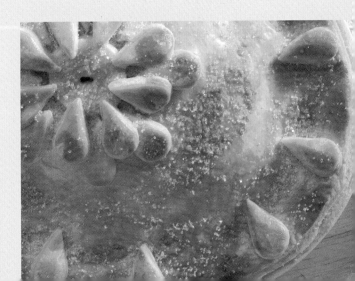

chocolate mousse

SERVES 4
COOKING TIME 5 MINUTES
(plus 30 minutes chilling time)

175g/6oz chocolate (at least 70% cocoa solids),
  in pieces
4 free-range eggs, separated

1 Put the chocolate in a heatproof bowl and place
   over a saucepan of boiling water until melted,
   stirring continuously. Be careful not to overheat
   the chocolate.
2 Allow the chocolate to cool, then beat in the
   egg yolks.
3 Whisk the egg whites until stiff, then carefully fold
   into the chocolate mixture. Spoon into a serving
   dish and chill for at least 30 minutes.

cherry toast

As a dessert or starter, this dish boosts the brain with
antioxidants and trace elements.

SERVES 4
COOKING TIME 10 MINUTES

40g/1½oz butter
Pinch ground cinnamon
1 teaspoon sugar or sucralose
1 French baguette, cut into 2.5cm/1in slices
225g/8oz cherries, stoned and halved
1 tablespoon flaked almonds

1 Mix the butter, cinnamon and sugar or sucralose
   and spread the mixture onto the bread.
2 Top with the cherries and place under a hot grill
   until the bread is golden brown. Garnish with
   almonds and serve immediately.

crème brûlée

As well as being a source of energy, the eggs in creme
brûlée give it proteins and lecithin. The liquorice root
can reduce levels of cortisone, the stress hormone, as
well as aiding premenstrual and menopausal symptoms.

SERVES 4
COOKING TIME 25 MINUTES
(plus 2 hours chilling time)

500ml/18fl oz skimmed milk
2 tablespoons sugar or sucralose
1 piece liquorice root
Zest of 1 lemon
4 free-range egg yolks
3 tablespoons brown sugar
1 tablespoon cornflour
1 tablespoon ground ginger
2 drops vanilla essence

1 Place the milk, sugar or sucralose, liquorice root
   and lemon zest in a saucepan and heat gently.
2 Whisk the egg yolks with 1 tablespoon of the brown
   sugar, the cornflour, ground ginger and vanilla
   essence in a large heatproof bowl. Gradually add
   the hot milk mixture, stirring all the time.
3 Return the mixture to the saucepan and bring to
   the boil. Reduce the heat and cook for 5 minutes,
   stirring continuously.
4 Pour into 4 ramekins, transfer to the fridge and chill
   for 2 hours.
5 Sprinkle the remaining brown sugar over the top
   of each ramekin, and place under a hot grill until
   the sugar begins to bubble. Chill for 10 minutes
   and serve.

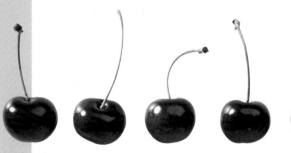

chocolate cake

It will be a great relief to many to hear that chocolate is packed with antioxidants and tryptophan!

SERVES 8
COOKING TIME 60 MINUTES

For the cake:
150g/5½oz salted butter
150g/5½oz unrefined brown muscovado sugar
3 medium free-range eggs, beaten
175g/6oz self-raising flour
Pinch of salt
Milk
2 tablespoons cocoa powder
2-3 drops vanilla essence

For the icing:
55g/2oz salted butter
175g/6oz icing sugar
2 tablespoons cocoa powder
Zest of 1 medium orange (optional)

1 Line the bottom of two deep 18cm/7in cake tins with buttered greaseproof paper. Cream the butter and muscovado sugar.
2 Gradually beat in the eggs, a little at a time. Then sieve the flour and salt gradually into the mixture, adding a little milk to keep it moist (the mixture should remain at a dripping consistency).
3 Stir in the cocoa powder and vanilla essence.
4 Spoon the mixture into the prepared cake tins. Spread it almost to the sides of the tins and leave a slight hollow in the middle for a more even rise.
5 Cook on the middle of the oven at 170°C for 25–30 minutes or until the sponge is light and springy and a skewer inserted into the cake comes out clean. Allow the cakes to cool in the tins for 5 minutes then turn out onto a cooling rack.
6 To make the icing, mix butter, icing sugar, cocoa powder and orange zest, if using.
7 Spread half the icing over the inner surface of one cake, and half over the outer surface of the other, and sandwich together, or simply share the icing over the two and enjoy them separately!

oranges with warm honey and walnuts

Since ancient times, honey has been known as a great source of sugar—but it is twice as sweet as sugar, so use less. It is rich in vitamins and is an antiseptic.

SERVES 4
COOKING TIME 20 MINUTES

4 large oranges, peeled
100g/3½oz clear honey
20 walnuts, peeled and roughly chopped
4 teaspoons Cointreau (optional)
Whipped cream or Greek yoghurt, to serve

1 Slice the oranges horizontally into 1cm/½in slices, retaining the shape of the orange, and place in individual dishes.
2 In a small saucepan, heat the honey over a low heat, stirring continuously.
3 Sprinkle the walnuts over the oranges and add a teaspoon of Cointreau (if using) to each orange.
4 Cover each orange with the warm honey and serve with cream or yoghurt.

index

acknowledgments

"Thank" is probably too weak a word; but we wish to thank our parents for unconditional support; our teachers and colleagues for stimulating our fascination with the brain and it's workings; our patients for reciprocating our interest in nutrition and the brain; Ian Wood for his editing skills, and Amy Carroll and Louise Dixon of our publishers for their faith and patience in helping us realize our dream.

Carroll & Brown Publishers would like to thank:

Production Manager Karol Davies
Computer Management Paul Stradling
Photographer's Assistant David Yems
Picture Research Sandra Schneider
Food Preparation Claire Lewis
Proofreader Geoffrey West
Indexer Madeline Weston

Picture credits
11 BSIP, Jacopin/SPL
12 (right) David Gifford/SPL
15 (bottom) Getty Images
18 Alfred Pasieka/SPL
26 (bottom) Getty Images
45 (bottom) William Gray/OSF
48 BSIP, Laurent/SPL
52 Getty Images
55 BSIP, Laurent/Laeticia/SPL
62 Alfred Pasieka/SPL
70 Getty Images
79 Getty Images
92 Getty Images
97 Roger Dixon